BASIC
PSYCHOPHARMACOLOGY

Alvin J. Levenson has lectured and written extensively on psychopharmacology and has over fifty publications to his credit. His pragmatic approach to the topic has earned him enthusiastic responses from numerous physician and non-physician health care specialties and disciplines. He received his M.D. from the University of Texas Medical Branch and did specialty training in psychiatry at Baylor College of Medicine and subspecialty training in gerontology and geriatrics at Texas Research Institute of Mental Sciences, both at the Texas Medical Center. He is in full-time academic medicine as Chief of the Section on Geriatric Psychiatry at The University of Texas Medical School at Houston and is a lecturer in Psychopharmacology and Aging at Baylor College of Medicine. He sits on national, county, and local policymaking committees and is Editor-in-Chief of *Gerontology and Geriatrics Education Journal*.

BASIC
PSYCHOPHARMACOLOGY

Alvin J. Levenson, M.D.

SPRINGER PUBLISHING COMPANY ■ NEW YORK

Springer Publishing Company, Inc.
200 Park Avenue South
New York, New York 10003

81 82 83 84 85 / 10 9 8 7 6 5 4 3 2 1

Library of Congress Cataloging in Publication Data

Levenson, Alvin J
    Basic psychopharmacology.

    Includes bibliographies and index.
    1. Psychopharmacology.   I.   Title.
    RM315.L45   615'.7882   80-22267
ISBN 0-8261-2680-4
ISBN 0-8261-2681-2 (pbk.)

Printed in the United States of America

Contents

Preface

The major goal of this text is to assist in improving the psychopharma-cotherapeutic techniques of students and graduate health professionals who have either a present or a future role in the prescription, administration, or monitoring of psychopharmacologic regimens. Having had the pleasant opportunity to lecture rather extensively on psychopharmacology to medical and nursing students; psychiatric residents; residents and practicing physicians from other specialities; and psychologists, social workers, and other health care professionals, I became aware very quickly of their intense interest in psychopharmacology. Not only were those prescribing psychopharmacological agents interested in learning more about the field, but large numbers of those responsible for monitoring others' prescriptions, most of whom felt a great void in their fund of knowledge, were eager to enhance their knowledge and skills as well. Audiences responded well to these lectures, feeling more comfortable with such information about this aspect of patient care. It is mainly in response to their requests that this book is written. Therefore, this text is intended not only for physicians or physicians-to-be but also for use in other disciplines playing a major role in health care delivery.

This book is not meant to be a comprehensive text, a cookbook approach to the topic, or a bible to the field. It is a teaching text, structuring, presenting, and emphasizing those principles and information that have been relatively well verified by research and clinical experience, and providing a bridge between these principles and information and clinical application. When more theoretical or less substantial concepts are addressed, they are represented as such; indeed, they are used only when they are relevant to a clinical approach. When less-well-documented ideas cannot be or are not applied in this way, I mean not to discredit them but rather to stimulate further investigative verification by the reader. I have tried to provide the reader with the most relevant sources; in some cases these sources are the original research in the area, augmented by current references.

Although mental illness is widespread, many psychopathological states are responsive to psychopharmacotherapy. However, in the hands of unlearned, unskilled, or casual practitioners, misuse of psychopharmacological agents can increase the risk of a nontherapeutic outcome. Incorrect selection of a drug—or selection of one when none is indicated—will produce no benefit to the patient, and may cause harm. Moreover, expecting these medications to be a panacea, unaccompanied by some form of psychotherapy, counseling, or environmental change, may disappoint physician and patient, and may threaten both the patient's recovery and the quality of the therapeutic relationship. When pharmacological control, rather than remission of the target clinical complex, is the major treatment goal, the best interests of the patient are not served. In cases in which careful starting dosages and target concentrations, adjusted for stature, age, bioequivalency, and disease state are not devised, or in which current physiologic status is not adequately known, potentially harmful agents may severely disrupt physiological homeostatis. This unfortunate outcome may worsen the patient's psychological status. Such outcomes are generally avoidable.

Psychopharmacology has the potential to be an exact science. A body of significant research findings, replicated in clinical settings, has removed much of the speculation from psychopharmacotherapy. From these findings emerges a general set of requirements for the optimal use of psychotropic medications. The health care professional must have:

1.   a working knowledge of psychopharmacologically responsive psychopathology—that is, the ability to recognize psychological symptoms and signs, either spontaneous or offered by the patient in response to specific questions that can identify the patient's potential responsiveness to the indicated class of psychotropic agents;

2.   a general understanding of pharmacokinetics (the fate of a drug after its administration) and pharmacodynamics (the effects of the drug);

3.   a working knowledge of each major psychotropic agent group, and specifically, the more commonly prescribed drugs in the group, pertinent pharmacokinetics, purported loci and mechanisms of action, principles of use (indications, contraindications; efficacy; starting, titration, end-point and maintenance dosages; and side effects);

4.   a rapid psychiatric assessment instrument permitting collection of psychiatric data and determination of psychopharmacologically responsive syndromes;

5.   an appreciation of the patient's physiological status: his or her history, a physical examination, and appropriate and complete laboratory screening.

In this book I have sought to provide an easy-to-use elaboration of these requirements. I hope that this knowledge will provide effective and efficient guidelines for an optimal psychopharmacotherapeutic technique.

I wish sincerely to thank my students, whose encouragement prompted this effort; Mrs. Lenita Stanley and Ms. Cheryl Schutter for typing the manuscript; Ms. Elizabeth Gammon and Ms. Sue Fox for their editorial assistance; William E. Fann, M.D., for serving as a significant mentor to me during my training, as well as for his critical review of the manuscript; and the members of the Springer Publishing Company for their enthusiasm, interest, and support.

Foreword

Psychopharmacological agents are the most widely prescribed, widely misprescribed, most frequently abused, and probably most advertised of all the pharmaceuticals available to the practicing clinician. They clearly occupy a role at or near the center of medical practice.

Psychoactive compounds properly prescribed have enabled some people who otherwise "could not make it through the day" to conduct their lives in a reasonably normal fashion without more intrusive therapeutic intervention. The major tranquilizers, or antipsychotic agents such as chlorpromazine, have brought about what many people call a third revolution in psychiatry through massive reductions in resident mental hospital population. On the basis of hospital admission and discharge rates and the growth of the mental hospital population, a survey in 1950 predicted that by 1960 the mental hospital population would be double its 1950 level. The antipsychotic phenothiazines were introduced to psychiatric practice in 1952 by Delay and Deniker in France and dramatically aborted this grim projection. In 1960 follow-up mental hospital surveys showed that the population had not only failed to double, but had actually been substantially reduced from its 1950 level. The benzodiazepine anxiolytics and tricyclic antidepressants have achieved nearly equivalent significance in the successful treatment of nonpsychotic psychiatric disorders.

Psychoactive pharmaceuticals are not the sole factor in improved mental health care, but many of the other important elements, such as the community psychiatry movement, the increased number of mental health professionals, the value of the activity and training therapies, and the refinement of psychotherapeutic modalities are probably in large degree dependent upon the development of effective psychiatric medications.

Patients who would otherwise require hospitalization are now appropriately treated as outpatients with combinations of medication and supportive therapy.

Psychoactive medications are also commonly prescribed to people suffering from physiological ailments with significant emotional accompaniments; anxiety and depression are frequent complications of extended physical illness, disability, chronic pain, or injury. A knowledge of the indications, the beneficial effects, and the deleterious effects of these compounds is therefore necessary for all physicians, including those in specialties other than psychiatry or general practice. Dr. Levenson has compiled an excellent text detailing those aspects of clinical psychopharmacology that physicians, nurses, and allied health personnel are likely to encounter in their daily work with medicated patients and those requiring medication. He has distilled a great deal of knowledge into a clinically manageable handbook with enough specificity and theoretical background to demonstrate the rational pharmacologic principles that underlie the actions and prescriptive usefulness of the most prominent psychotropic agents. I commend this volume to health practitioners as a readable educational text and as a well-designed reference manual for the office or clinic.

William E. Fann, M.D.

CHAPTER 1

An Overview of Psychopharmacologically Responsive Psychiatric States

Psychopathology may be described as either functional or nonfunctional. Many of these states are responsive to the appropriate class of psychopharmacologic agents (see Chapters 3–6) and indicated form of psychotherapy, counseling, and/or environmental intervention.

Functional disorders are states that have no known organic etiology. Current research indicates, however, that certain of these conditions are associated with physiochemical abnormalities in the brain. For example, schizophrenia is linked with an elevation of brain dopamine (see Chapter 3). Reductions in brain dopamine, norepinephrine (serotonin) and 5-hydroxytryptamine are concomitants to certain depressions (see Chapter 5). It is interesting to note that psychotropic agents that correct these physiochemical abnormalities often ameliorate the clinical manifestations of the acute state, and may reduce the incidence of its recurrence. These issues will be reviewed more fully in subsequent chapters.

Nonfunctional disorders are states that are caused by specific pathologic conditions that may arise either within the brain (direct causes) or extracerebrally (indirect causes). Although the mechanisms of production are not known conclusively, the impairment has to do with disruption of cerebral neurons responsible for maintenance of adequate psychological function. Examples of causes of nonfunctional disorders include: tumors (benign or malignant; if malignant, primary or metastatic); trauma (e.g., head trauma producing an intracranial hemorrhage or trauma to other parts of the body that might produce blood loss sufficient to impair brain function); toxins, either inherently toxic (e.g., some illicit drugs, ethanol, methanol, heavy metals) or toxic because of excessive dosage or idiosyncratic or cumulative effects (e.g., arising from some combination of medications). Other frequently recognized causes of nonfunctional psychopathology include infection in the brain (e.g., abscess, encephalitis, or meningitis); infection in other parts of the body that adversely affects brain function (e.g., a pneumonia that reduces oxygen supply to the brain); degenerative brain disease (e.g., Alzheimer's, Pick's or senile degenerative brain disease, Huntington's chorea, Jacob-Creutzfeldt disease, multiple sclerosis); metabolic disorder (e.g., hypo- or hyperthyroidism, diabetes mellitus, renal dysfunction, congestive heart failure); disease of the cerebral blood vessels reducing blood and oxygen supply to critical brain areas (e.g., atherosclerosis, A-V malformations, collagen vascular disease); and hydrocephalus.

The various origins of nonfunctional disorders are elaborated here because of the implications for treatment: the proper initial clinical approach is detection and reversal of the organic cause rather than symptomatic relief with psychopharmacologic agents.

Importantly, functional and nonfunctional disorders often display many of the same characteristics, but certain features can signal the presence of a nonfunctional disorder. An obvious signal is a history of physiological evaluation suggesting an organic cause. Other signals are delusions and/or hallucinations that are frightening to the patient, although these may occur in functional disorders as well; visual, gustatory, olfactory, tactile, or kinesthetic hallucinations; or a psychiatric syndrome concurrent with an organic brain syndrome.[1]

Psychotropic agents may from time to time be indicated in treatment of a nonfunctional disorder if the disorder is potentially responsive, if a reversible cause cannot be identified, or if psychological suffering or a life-threatening situation is revealed. In such instances it is always wise to consult appropriate nonpsychiatric medical specialists to determine that a given drug is physiologically acceptable for a particular patient and to determine special physiologic monitoring techniques.

---

[1]The signs suggesting the diagnosis of organic brain syndrome include any of the following:
1. partial or total disorientation to time, place, and/or person;
2. partial or total loss of recent memory;
3. a greater-than-two-digit gap between the numbers that the patient can remember forward versus reversed (e.g., the patient can repeat "973201" exactly as given, but cannot correctly repeat at least four of these digits in reverse order);
4. impairment of intellectual function, including commonly known and general information (e.g., current president of United States) and simple calculations (e.g., 100 minus 7);
5. concrete thought processes, as described for manifest schizophrenia;
6. lability (excessive emotional expression with minimal or no provocation) or flat affect.

INDICATORS OF PSYCHOPHARMACOLOGICAL RESPONSIVENESS

Whether organic causes are present or absent, psychiatric states that are potentially responsive to medication have recognizable essential features in the clinical situation. Whatever the history or other clinical data may suggest, psychopharmacological decisions ideally should rest on these observed key symptoms and/or signs. These responsive states are outlined as follows (Freedman et al., 1975; Klein & Davis, 1969).

I. *Delusion*. A fixed, persistent, false belief that is unaffected by logical persuasion. (Note that this does not apply to beliefs that are rooted in patient's culture or life-style.) The most commonly occurring types of delusions are:

   A. *Paranoid*.

      1. Paranoid persecutory: Patient feels threatened and in potential danger from some source.

      2. Paranoid grandiose: Patient believes he or she possesses some special and unusual powers or occupies some exalted position or station in life.

   B. *Ideas of influence*. Patient believes that some outside power or force is controlling his or her mind, body, or actions.

   C. *Ideas of reference*. Patient believes that incidents occurring in the environment refer specifically to him or her.

   D. *Somatic*. Patient believes that something of a nonbizarre, physical nature is wrong with his or her body.

   E. *Nihilistic*. Patient believes that part or all of his or her body is being destroyed by some bizarre process, and/or that he or she no longer exists or has died.

   F. *Guilty*. Patient feels as though he or she has committed some unpardonable sin or crime.

II. *Hallucination*. A false sensory perception without a concrete external stimulus. They may be:

   A. Auditory.

   B. Visual.

   C. Tactile.

   D. Olfactory.

   E. Kinesthetic.

   F. Gustatory.

III. *Manifest schizophrenia*. May exist in various clinical subtypes producing variations in the presentation. The main symptoms or signs indicating the diagnosis ("primary" symptoms or signs), irrespective of the presence of delusions and/or hallucinations,[2] are:

A. *Disordered thought processes,* manifested by:
1. Blocking: Patient, presumably involuntarily, ceases thought and verbal productions, often in the middle of a thought or sentence.
2. Circumstantiality: Patient has a great deal of difficulty, if not total failure, in communicating a clear train of thought in expressing a central idea and, instead, tends to include much irrelevant data.
3. Tangentiality: Patient, in spontaneous renderings or in response to questions, offers totally irrelevant remarks.
4. Looseness of associations. Patient constructs sentences with unrelated or slightly related ideas, and does not indicate an intention to change the subject or explain the transition from one thought or phrase to the other.
5. Concreteness of thought processes: Patient is unable to generalize and abstract concrete verbal stimuli.

B. *Flat and/or inappropriate affect.* Patient exhibits an affect (external representation of mood) inappropriate for the thought(s) being expressed.

C. *Extreme ambivalence.* Patient is ambivalent toward almost everything, with the extremes of these ambivalent feelings in almost equal contest with each other.

D. *Autism.* Patient displays extremely subjective and self-centered thought; fantasy and daydreaming substitute for reality. Patient tends to apply private and personal meanings to situations and words, rather than consensually validated ones. He or she tends to be self-absorbed and preoccupied with stimuli from his or her internal world, often to the total or near-total exclusion of external stimuli.

IV. *Incipient psychosis.* Syndromes approaching manifest psychosis, but not yet psychotic, include two major types:

A. *Incipient schizophrenia,* characterized by:
1. Feeling of incomprehensible dread: Patient experiences a vague and unfounded feeling that something ominous is going to happen.
2. Tendency to react to seemingly minor events, previously

---

[2]This description of manifest schizophrenia (Section IIIA to D) is based on the Bleulerian primary criteria. Delusions and/or hallucinations (Bleulerian secondary criteria) are not specific to the diagnosis of manifest schizophrenia; they may accompany many other psychotic syndromes as well.

accepted with indifference or equanimity, as now specifically important and personally relevant.

3. Atypical eccentric concerns of the patient about the relationship of the world, universe, or "cosmos" to self.

4. Depersonalization: Patient often describes a feeling of unreality concerning the self—a feeling that some parts of the body, especially the brain or "mind," have changed size or proportion to others.

5. Derealization: Patient feels that the environment or the people and/or objects in it have somehow changed and no longer seem real.

6. Preoccupation with religious or philosophical ideas: Patient is atypically attendant to these ideas.

B. *Incipient delusion*. The beginnings of ideation characterized at its maturity by one of the divisions in section I.

V. *Depression*. The common psychopharmacologically responsive depressions are:

A. *Retarded type*. Patient exhibits a reduction in overall motility and verbal production, a depressed mood or affect, a deceleration in the rate and amplitude of thought production, and/or depressive thought content (may or may not be accompanied by incipient or manifest schizophrenia, incipient or manifest delusions, or hallucinations).

B. *Anxious type*. Patient displays symptoms and/or signs of varying severities of anxiety (the most severe being agitation), as well as depression (including subjective complaints, a depressed affect, and/or depressive thought content). Features that are helpful in corroborating this diagnosis are an accompanying initial and/or intermittent sleep disturbance and depression that is worse in the afternoon and/or evening, is continuous and essentially without change in severity throughout the day, or occurs in response to situations (may or may not be accompanied by incipient or manifest schizophrenia, incipient or manifest delusions, or hallucinations).

C. *Mixed type*. Patient displays a combination of the retarded and anxious types.

VI. *Acute mania*. The key clinical components of this syndrome include an overall increase in motor activity, an increased amplitude (pressure) of speech, an elated affect, rapid and shifting thought production (flight of ideas),[3] an increased amplitude (pressure) of thought,

---

[3] In contrast to "looseness of associations" (see section III, A.4), the patient manifesting flight of ideas logically orders his or her phrases or sentences.

and grandiose thought content. Mania may not be accompanied by incipient or manifest schizophrenia, incipient or manifest delusions, or hallucinations.

VII. *Acute hypomania*. This syndrome is manifested by the same symptoms or signs as in mania, but of lesser intensity. As with acute mania, hypomania may be accompanied by incipient or manifest schizophrenia, incipient or manifest delusions, or hallucinations.

REFERENCES

Freedman, A. M., Kaplan, H. I., and Sadock, B. J. (eds.). *Comprehensive Textbook of Psychiatry* (Vols. I, II). Williams and Wilkins, Baltimore, 1975.
Klein, D. F., and Davis, J. M. *Diagnosis and Drug Treatment of Psychiatric Disorders*. Williams and Wilkins, Baltimore, 1969.

CHAPTER 2

An Overview
of Drug Action

Medications are prescribed to correct, or assist in correcting, a specified abnormality usually occurring in a particular structure or set of structures of the body. To produce optimal therapeutic effect, a drug must reach the target structure(s) in sufficient quantity to produce the desired change without acting on nontarget structures or producing unwanted and ill effects. Unfortunately, most medications are not so specific as to affect only target structures. For example, a patient with complaints of abdominal pain sees a physician. After careful study, the physician diagnoses the patient's pain as resulting from stomach ulcers. Part of the treatment consists of a medication that slows down the stomach's activity to reduce the secretion of the ulcer-causing acid. Prescribed in the appropriate dosage, the medication not only reduces the activity of the stomach, but, as an extension of its desired effects, also reduces the motility of the esophagus (causing nausea) and of the large intestine (producing constipation). Additionally, this drug affects the brain, disturbing cognition and memory, and it causes an acceleration of heart rate.

It is admittedly unusual for a drug to produce such severe and multiple side effects. This situation is more likely to occur either when the medication is prescribed in excessive dosage or when the patient's current physical condition predisposes him or her to such insult.

PHARMACOKINETIC PROCESSES

Before and after any drug's action on the target receptor sites, there are numerous normally occurring processes (pharmacokinetics) that are essential to its therapeutic effect. These pharmacokinetic processes include the

7

manner and rate of absorption of the drug into the bloodstream; its circulation to and concentration in the various target organs; its breakdown, or metabolism, into an inactive state; and its excretion or elimination from the body.

Absorption and Circulation

For a medication administered by mouth, the initial step in the pharmacokinetic process is absorption through the cells of the gastrointestinal lining, the mucosa, into the bloodstream. In order to pass through the mucosal cells, the drug must be in a form that permits it to cross the cell membranes and enter the cells themselves. To permeate cell membranes, which are composed largely of lipids (fats), the medication must be soluble in water or in lipids. With the exception of lithium, all psychotropic agents are lipid soluble, and diffuse passively into the intestinal cells. (Lithium moves across the cell membrane by a process known as active transport, which involves the movement of the drug by its association with a specific component of the membrane. "Active" indicates an energy-dependent process not automatically occurring in the absence of special requirements.)

Another requirement for passage of the drug across the cell membrane is its degree of ionization. Medications are compounds, that is, composed of two or more elements (an element being a particle that cannot be broken down further). In order for the compound to hold together, each element must have an electrical charge, and the number of positive charges must equal the number of negative charges in the compound. Ionization is the dissociation of the compound into its component charged elements (ions). Nonionized compounds are far more lipid soluble than ionized compounds, so their uptake and passage across the cell membrane are more rapid. The acidity (pH) of the gastrointestinal contents plays a role in determining the amount of ionization, the more acidic (lower pH) being less ionized and, hence more lipid soluble.

From the intestinal mucosa, a drug is absorbed into the smaller blood vessels, thence into general circulation, and ultimately to the target receptors. Some medications, such as psychotropic agents, are believed to exert their predominant therapeutic action in the brain. In order to reach the brain, medications must penetrate the blood-brain barrier, a group of microscopic structures that protect the cerebrum from many noxious substances. Interestingly, nonionized (lipid-soluble) compounds are able to reach the brain tissues.

The rate of absorption of a drug and the amount that reaches the general circulation are called its bioavailability, indicating the availability of the drug to act at the target receptor sites. Different drugs and different forms of the same drug vary in their degree of bioavailability. For example, if the medication is administered parenterally (intramuscularly, sub-cutaneously, or intravenously), it bypasses the gastrointestinal tract and liver (which is a major obstacle to bioavailability because it is the body's major metabolic organ for most drugs) and achieves more rapid circulation than when it is administered orally. The equivalence of drugs and their various forms—the amount of each required to achieve the desired level of concentration in the target organs—will be discussed, for each drug group, in Chapters 3–6.

Blood proteins have the capacity to bind (combine with) nonprotein substances, including many drugs, usually in a reversible reaction. Drugs also vary in the proportion that can be bound (in the blood or other tissues).

Under ideal circumstances, an equilibrium should be established between the amount of a drug in its free active form available to act at receptor sites and the amount stored in tissues for future use. Influencing this equilibrium is the quantity of medication bound to blood protein. Any decrease in protein binding may significantly increase the amount of free active drug. For example, if only 6% of a drug is normally bound, a decrement in binding, even though small, may actually double the amount of the drug available for action on receptor sites.

Metabolism and Excretion

The breakdown, or metabolism, of a pharmacologically active compound into an inactive state occurs primarily in the liver, although the compound also may be converted to other active substances in that organ.

Were active substances and their breakdown products to remain indef-initely in circulation, the risk of adverse effects would increase. Therefore, medications must be eliminated from the body at a rate sufficient to avoid toxic levels. The standard measure of the body's elimination rate is called the half-life of a drug, which is the time required for the body to eliminate one half of that drug present in the system at the point when measurement was begun. Stated another way, it is the time needed for a given level in the blood to decline to one-half of the value first measured.

Elimination of most drugs occurs via the kidneys into the urine. Active lipid-soluble drugs are converted into inactive water-soluble substances, allowing excretion in the urine (Fingl & Woodbury, 1975; Friedel, 1978; Hollister, 1979). Adequate renal function is required for adequate excre-tion of the converted agents.

NEUROLOGICAL PRINCIPLES

A basic familiarity with certain neurological principles is necessary for an understanding of both the intended effects and many side effects of psychotropic medications on therapeutic target receptors within the brain. For introductory purposes, neuroanatomy and neurophysiology can be summarized as follows.

Neuroanatomy

The nervous system includes two major parts: the central nervous system (CNS) and the peripheral nervous system (PNS) (see Figure 2–1). The central nervous system consists of the brain and the spinal cord. The peripheral nervous system is composed of the spinal nerves (31 pairs arising from the spinal cord, one of each pair for the right side and the other for the left side of the body) and the cranial nerves (12 pairs arising from the brain, one of each pair for the right side and the other for the left side of the body).

The PNS has two major functions: motor and sensory. The motor fibers are of two types: somatic and autonomic. The somatic nerve fibers carry motor impulses from the spinal cord to the skeletal muscles. The autonomic fibers, which are carried within the cranial or spinal nerves, are of either the sympathetic or parasympathetic type, and supply motor innervation to most of the body's organs. Together, the sympathetic and parasympathetic autonomic nerves, and the structures from which they arise in the brain, are called the autonomic nervous system (ANS).

The sympathetic autonomic nerves arising from the spinal cord are called preganglionic and are, in essence, presynaptic neurons; they end in the sympathetic trunk just outside the spinal cord. The postganglionic, or postsynaptic sympathetic neurons, arise in the sympathetic trunk, and end on certain structures, supplying motor innervation to them. Numerous organs receive this motor innervation; the most pertinent ones affected by psychotropic medications are the heart and arterial blood vessels. The normal sympathetic effect on these structures is acceleration of heart rate, augmentation of force of heart contraction, and constriction of the arterial blood vessels.

The preganglionic or presynaptic parasympathetic nerves arise from two major origins: certain of the cranial nerves and the spinal nerves arising from the cord's sacral portion. The postganglionic, or postsynaptic, parasympathetic nerves arise from the presynaptic parasympathetic neuron. Those arising from the cranial portion furnish motor innervation to the

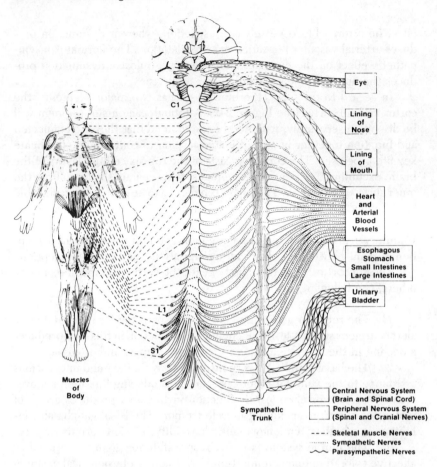

Eye

Lining of Nose

Lining of Mouth

Heart and Arterial Blood Vessels

Esophagous Stomach Small Intestines Large Intestines

Urinary Bladder

C1

T1

L1

S1

Muscles of Body

Sympathetic Trunk

Central Nervous System (Brain and Spinal Cord)
Peripheral Nervous System (Spinal and Cranial Nerves)

---- Skeletal Muscle Nerves
.... Sympathetic Nerves
⌇⌇ Parasympathetic Nerves

Figure 2–1.   POSTERIOR VIEW OF CENTRAL AND PERIPHERAL NERVOUS SYSTEM

following structures that often are affected by psychotropic drugs: the eye (constriction of the pupil); nose (mucus secretion); mouth (salivary gland secretion); heart (reduction in heart rate); the esophagus, stomach, small and large intestines (peristalsis, or regular and rhythmical contractions moving food through and out of the gastrointestinal tract); and the bladder (contraction to produce emptying). Any lesion or chemical dysfunction at the origin of the autonomic nervous system in the brain or along the peripheral sympathetic or parasympathetic presynaptic, synaptic, or post-synaptic levels can produce abnormalities that assume the form opposite to the intended physiological effect. For example, the normal sympathetic effect on arterial blood vessels is constriction, whereas dysfunction produces arterial vascular relaxation or vasodilatation. The normal parasympathetic effect on the eye constricts the pupil (miosis); dysfunction produces the opposite effect (dilatation, or mydriasis).

In regard to the CNS, the brain itself has two major segments: the cortex and subcortex (see Figure 2–2). Although each major segment will be discussed separately, it should be understood that they are connected and function together in a coordinated fashion to control and coordinate key life processes. The cortex consists of the top six cellular layers of the brain, excluding the linings, or meninges, that separate the brain from the inner surface of the skull. The cortex is believed to be primarily responsible for intellect, judgment, affective stability, forebearance, fine and gross motor function, horizontal eye movements, speech, voluntary and involuntary urination and defecation, memory, auditory perception, perception of pain, light touch, temperature sensations, and visual perception.

The subcortical structures lie beneath the cortex and include, among others, the following.

1. The reticular activating system is responsible for maintaining an alert conscious state. A lesion or chemical dysfunction in this area produces a decline in the level of alertness—lethargy, stupor, and/or coma.

2. The basal ganglia are responsible for involuntary and unconscious assistance to the voluntary motor system in producing fine motor movements. A lesion or chemical dysfunction in this area produces a lack of motor coordination, including muscle tremor. The basal ganglia also inhibit an involuntary tendency to muscle rigidity; a lesion permits rigidity.

3. The limbic system is partly responsible for giving emotional or affective coloration to incoming stimuli. A lesion or physiological dysfunction produces a range of abnormal psychological or behavioral phenomena.

4. The hypothalamus, among other functions, serves as the seat of the autonomic nervous system, which controls motor activity of the hollow viscera (the heart and blood vessels, lungs, gastrointestinal tract, etc.). A lesion or chemical dysfunction produces an impairment of visceral function.

5. The hypothalamic-pituitary axis controls endocrine hormonal secretion in the body. A lesion or dysfunction produces abnormally elevated or reduced hormonal secretion and consequent physiological dysfunction.

Only those subcortical structures theorized either to be implicated in the production of certain psychiatric disturbances or to be affected by various psychotropic agents are briefly listed and described. Other key

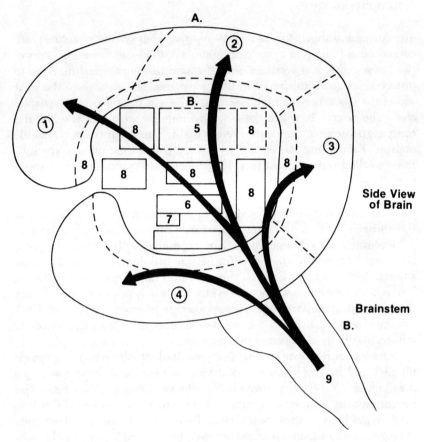

A. Cerebral Cortex   B. Cerebral Sub-Cortex
   1. Frontal Lobe   5. Basal Ganglia
   2. Parietal Lobe   6. Hypothalamus
   3. Occipital Lobe   7. Hypothalamic-Pituitary Axis
   4. Temporal Lobe   8. Components of Limbic System
                                          9. Reticular Activating System

Figure 2–2.   CORTEX AND SUBCORTEX (LONGITUDINAL SECTION)

subcortical structures include the cerebellum (involved in unconscious motor coordination) and thalamus (important to transmission of pain, light touch, and temperature sensations to the cortex, unconscious motor control, smell, limbic system function, and maintenance of an alert state).

Neurophysiology

The cortex and subcortex, as well as other nervous system structures, are composed of billions of nerve cells (neurons), the basic functional units of the brain and spinal cord. In order for normal neurological function to proceed, an electrical impulse must pass from one neuron to the next across the space between the neurons, known as the synapse or synaptic cleft. The neuron in which the electrical impulse originates is called the presynaptic neuron; the neuron receiving the impulse is the postsynaptic neuron. Facilitating the excitation of the postsynaptic neuron are substances called neurotransmitters. These chemicals, synthesized and stored in presynaptic neurons, are released into the synaptic cleft on stimulation by the electrical impulse (see Figure 2-3).

The neurotransmitters believed to play a significant role in neural transmission within the brain (primarily subcortically) include norepinephrine and its chemical precursor, dopamine (both known as catecholamines); acetylcholine; serotonin (an indoleamine); and gamaaminobutyric acid, or GABA. These neurotransmitters are distributed throughout the brain, each neuron synthesizing only one substance, so that there are norepinephrine neurons, dopamine neurons, and so on. Continuing research is likely to disclose the existence of additional neurotransmitters and their actions and interactions.

Once a neurotransmitter has been secreted into the synapse or synaptic cleft and has acted on the postsynaptic neuron, at least two major possibilities exist with respect to its fate (see Figure 2-4). First, the neurotransmitter may be metabolized (destroyed or broken down into inactive products) in the synaptic cleft. This is the case with small amounts of catecholamines (dopamine and norepinphrine), and is a principal means of acetylcholine destruction. The second fate, and the one believed to be the major route of inactivation for dopamine, norepinephrine, serotonin, and GABA, is that they are taken up again into the respective presynaptic neurons, where they are either reaggregated into storage vesicles for later secretion, or metabolized by an enzyme. The intraneuronal enzyme responsible for degrading the catecholamines and serotonin is monoamine oxidase (MAO); and for GABA, it is believed to be GABA-T (Guyton, 1976; Iverson, 1978; Snyder, 1972).

Because much of normal psychological function is mediated by the brain, neurotransmitter abnormalities are believed to play a prominent role in the biogenesis of certain psychiatric states. These will be discussed more fully in Chapters 3-6.

Throughout Chapters 3-5 the reader will see the terms anticholinergic, alpha adrenolytic (or alpha receptor blocking), and antidopa-

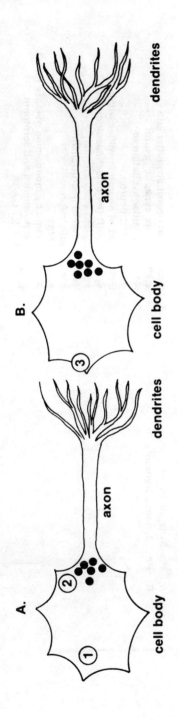

A. **Pre-Synaptic Neuron**
B. **Post-Synaptic Neuron**

1. Inhibition of electrical impulse in pre-synaptic neuron
2. Impulse activates emptying of neurotramsmitter storage vessicles into synapse
3. Neurotramsmitter activates post-synaptic neuron at which point the process begins again.

Figure 2–3. REPRESENTATION OF NEURONAL EXCITATION

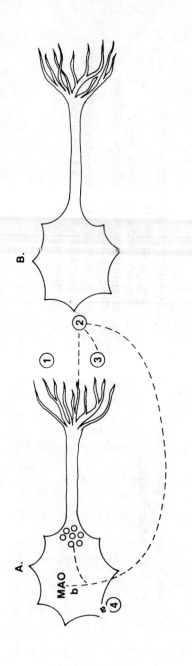

A. Pre-Synaptic Neuron
B. Post-Synaptic Neuron

1. Secretion of neurotransmitter into cleft from pre-synaptic neuron
2. Neurotransmitter excitation of post-synaptic neuron
3. Destruction of neurotransmitter within synaptic cleft (for catecholamines, serotonin, and acetylcholine)
4. Reabsorption of neurotransmitter into pre-synaptic neuron;
   a. re-storage
   b. destruction by monoamine oxidase (MAO for catecholamines and serotonin, GABA-T for GABA

Figure 2–4. NEUROTRANSMITTER FATE AFTER SECRETION INTO SYNAPTIC CLEFT AND EXCITATION OF POSTSYNAPTIC RECEPTOR

16

minergic describing substances or effects. The prefix anti and the suffix lytic, in these cases, indicate blocking; for example, anticholinergic means the blocking of acetylcholine, adrenolytic signifies the blocking of adrenaline (epinephrine) or an adrenaline-like substance (e.g., norepinephrine), and antidopaminergic specifies the blocking of dopamine.

In most cases, this blocking of a neurotransmitter occurs at the postsynaptic neuron, via a process called competitive inhibition. This process can be understood by visualizing the postsynaptic neuron as having receptor sites upon which the neurotransmitter acts after binding itself to these sites. For the neurotransmitter to be bound to the receptor, its molecules must conform in some way to the structure of the receptor site. In competitive inhibition, some molecule, usually chemically similar to or mimicking the substance that ordinarily acts on the postsynaptic receptor, competes with the regular substance for receptor sites. When a sufficient quantity of receptor sites have been occupied by the competitor, the normal physiological effect of the regular substance is interrupted or inhibited. If the consequent physiological dysfunction is unintended, nontherapeutic, and clinically manifest, it is known as a side effect.

Anticholinergic

Any substance that blocks the action of acetylcholine on its postsynaptic receptor site is known as anticholinergic. Acetylcholine is the neurotransmitter responsible for mediating electrical activation of the postsynaptic receptors of both the sympathetic and parasympathetic portions of the autonomic nervous system (ANS). Furthermore, it is the neurotransmitter that mediates activation of the end organs of the parasympathetic portion. Any compound that has sufficient anticholinergic potential will block those functions. For example, it is known that the parasympathetic nervous system, via acetylcholine secretions, maintains normal peristalsis of the intestine and contraction of the bladder. An anticholinergic substance could reduce intestinal peristalsis, cause constipation and reduce bladder contraction, resulting in impaired expulsion of urine from the bladder into the urethra, making it more difficult to void (urinary hesitancy, or in more severe cases, urinary retention). It is known that the sympathetic portion of the ANS mediates constriction of arterial blood vessels, permitting a blood pressure sufficient to move blood throughout the arterial network and bring nourishment to the various tissues of the body. Because acetylcholine is required for activation of the postsynaptic neurons that end on the arterial blood vessels, an anticholinergic substance could reduce sympathetic activity and diminish vascular constriction, causing a lowered arterial blood pressure (hypotension).

Alpha and Beta Blocking

The structures that are innervated by the postsynaptic sympathetic neurons have two basic types of receptor sites: alpha and beta. Activation of alpha receptors results in constriction of arterial blood vessels (vasoconstriction). Beta stimulation produces an increase in heart rate and force of cardiac contraction. The principal neurotransmitters mediating alpha and beta receptor stimulation are two of the three catecholamines, epinephrine and norepinephrine; the latter is primarily responsible for vasoconstriction. An alpha blocking agent is one that blocks the action of the appropriate neurotransmitter on the alpha receptors; a beta blocking agent interferes with the action of catecholamines on the beta receptors. Both actions are known as sympatholytic, that is resulting in an interruption of the usual sympathetic response. For example, the beta sympatholytic response yields a reduction in heart rate and force of cardiac contraction (also potentially producing a reduction in blood pressure, because less blood is pumped per heart beat). An agent with alpha blocking properties interferes with the action of norepinephrine with a consequent reduction in arterial blood pressure. Any substance resembling or mimicking the sympathetic effect is called a sympathomimetic agent.

Antidopaminergic

Any substance that blocks the action of dopamine at its postsynaptic receptor site is known as antidopaminergic. In addition to the role of dopamine in certain psychiatric states, the key activity of this neurotransmitter is its mediation of normal basal ganglia function. Dopamine blocking at the level of the basal ganglia likely will produce certain clinical manifestations such as Parkinson's disease and other abnormal motor movements, such as acute dystonias and dyskinesias, as well as akathisia (see Chapters 3 and 8). A reduction of brain dopamine concentration has been implicated in all of these.

REFERENCES

Fingl, E., and Woodbury, D. M. General Principles, in L. S. Goodman and A. Gillman (eds.), *The Pharmacological Basis of Therapeutics*, 5th ed. Macmillan, New York, 1975, pp. 1–46.

Friedel, R. O. Pharmacokinetics in the Geropsychiatric Patient, in M. A. Lipton, A. DiMascio, and K. F. Killam (eds.), *Psychopharmacy: A Generation of Progress*. Raven Press, New York, 1978, pp. 1499–1506.

Guyton, A. C. *Structure and Function of the Nervous System*. W. B. Saunders, Philadelphia, 1976.

Hollister, L. E. Psychotherapeutic Drugs, in A. Levenson (ed.), *Neuropsychiatric Side Effects of Drugs in the Elderly*. Raven Press, New York, 1979.

Iverson, L. L. Biochemical Pharmacology of GABA, in M. A. Lipton, A. DiMascio, and K. F. Killam (eds.), *Psychopharmacology: A Generation of Progress*. Raven Press, New York, 1978, pp. 26–27.

Snyder, S. H. Catecholamines and Serotonin, in R. W. Albers, G. J. Siegel, R. Katzman, and B. W. Agranoff (eds.), *Basic Neurochemistry*. Little, Brown, Boston, 1972, pp. 89–104.

CHAPTER 3

Major Tranquilizers

Major tranquilizers, as a class of psychotropic medications, sometimes are referred to by other names: ataractics, neuroleptics, antischizophrenics, antipsychotics. None of these alternative labels is adequate. For example, an ataractic produces peace or calmness of mind, but other psychotropic agent groups have the identical effect. A neuroleptic exerts its predominant action at the level of the central nervous system, but other classes of medication are believed to do so as well. Thus, drug effect does not distinguish this class. Major tranquilizers are indeed the drugs of choice for schizophrenia, but schizophrenia is only one of many types of psychosis in which they are efficacious. Finally, although major tranquilizers are antipsychotics for some psychoses, other psychotropic groups are effective for other psychoses. Therefore, it seems that none of the alternative names are completely useful and that "major tranquilizers" may be the best term for this group just because the term is nondescript.

COMMONLY USED MAJOR TRANQUILIZERS

Table 3–1 lists the commonly prescribed major tranquilizers in the United States. Major tranquilizers and phenothiazines traditionally have been used interchangeably, but phenothiazines are only one of five subgroups of the major tranquilizers. Those listed in Table 3–1 are available in their solid forms (tablet or capsule); most are available in the liquid or concentrate form, many in the intramuscularly administered fast-acting salt form, and only one (fluphenazine decanoate, Prolixin®), in an intramuscularly administered long-acting compound. Chlorpromazine and prochlorperazine can be secured in suppository form.

Table 3–1
Commonly Prescribed Major Tranquilizers

Phenothiazines
Aliphatic subgroup
chlorpromazine (Thorazine, CPZ)
Piperidine subgroup
thioridazine (Mellaril®)
mesoridazine (Serentil®)
Piperazine subgroup
acetophenazine (Tindal®)
prochlorperazine (Compazine®)
perphenazine (Trilafon®)
trifluoperazine (Stelazine®)
fluphenazine (Prolixin®)
Thioxanthenes
thiothixene (Navane®)
chlorprothixene (Taractan®)
Butyrophenone
haloperidol (Haldol®)
Dibenzoxazepine
loxapine succinate (Loxitane®)
Dihydroindolone
molindone (Moban®)

PERTINENT PHARMACOKINETICS

Major tranquilizers in the oral solid form are absorbed through the intestinal mucosa, at a rate varying from one person to another and in response to the concomitant administration of other drugs (e.g., antacids, which may reduce the completeness of absorption) (Fann et al., 1973). This form yields peak blood concentrations in approximately 1.5–3 hours (Hollister et al., 1970; Groves & Mandell, 1975). The liquid or concentrate form tends to be absorbed less erratically. Intramuscularly administered major tranquilizers move directly into the bloodstream (bypassing the gut and liver) and attain a peak blood level almost immediately after injection.

Regardless of the route of administration, once in the bloodstream these agents' pH, low ionization, high lipophilic (lipid soluble) nature, and high protein binding favor their absorption and uptake into tissues. In addition to crossing the blood-brain barrier, they enter most other tissues of the body. However, they seem to concentrate especially in the pulmonary tissues and in keratin-containing tissues such as hair, skin, and nails (Forrest et al., 1968).

With one major exception, major tranquilizers are metabolized primarily by the liver. The one exception is loxapine succinate (Loxitane®), which is metabolized primarily by the kidneys (Moyano, 1975). Approximately one-third of an administered dose of major tranquilizers is excreted via the urine in a 24-hour period; ultimately almost all the metabolites of the major tranquilizers are eliminated via this route. Although the half-life of major tranquilizers is relatively short, their duration of action is sufficiently long to permit a once-a-day administration with at least a 24-hour duration of therapeutic action.

THEORIES CONCERNING TRANQUILIZER ACTION

To understand some of the purported loci and mechanisms of action of major tranquilizers, it may be helpful to consider certain biochemical or biophysiological theories of the major tranquilizer-responsive states. This approach will provide a rationale for understanding how these agents assist in effecting a therapeutic response.

Several biological theories explain the etiology of schizophrenia. First, the essential problems are thought to occur at the subcortical level of the brain. Second, elevated levels of biogenic amines in the brain, notably dopamine, have been implicated (McGeer, 1971; Horn & Snyder, 1971; Snyder et al., 1974). Third, whether or not caused by elevated cerebral dopamine levels, there may be a hyperactive cerebral subcortical neuronal state. Fourth, some researchers have theorized that the schizophrenic individual is bombarded by a huge number of incoming stimuli via the reticular activating system, and that the quantity of these stimuli is sufficiently large to exceed the person's capacity to integrate them successfully (Mednick, 1958; Meehl, 1962). In addition, these incoming stimuli receive their emotional or affective charge from the limbic system.

Other psychoses have not been so completely studied as has schizophrenia. However, altered central nervous system biogenic amine levels have been implicated in the origins of some psychoses, especially the pharmacologically induced psychoses, for many of which major tranquilizers have been shown to be efficacious (Snyder et al., 1974). For example, amphetamines in sufficient dosage have been shown to produce a syndrome closely resembling paranoid schizophrenia as well as an acute paranoid persecutory state (without symptoms or signs of schizophrenia). Major tranquilizers are believed to exert their predominant therapeutic action at subcortical sites in the brain, at the cellular and structure or organ/system levels.

At least three theories place the therapeutic action of major tranquilizers at the cellular level. One theory suggests that these pharmacological compounds inhibit oxidative phosphorylation, causing a consequent decrease in cellular energy production. A second theory states that major tranquilizers combine with the cerebral subcortical neuronal membrane to decrease excitability. A third theory, currently the most commonly accepted, is that these agents, via competitive inhibition, block dopamine (as well as the other biogenic amines: norepinephrine and serotonin) at the level of the postsynaptic neuron; that is, the molecules of the tranquilizers compete with the neurotransmitters for receptor sites in the postsynaptic receptors (Burt et al., 1976). This theory has clinical relevance because both catecholamines and indoleamines have been implicated in the production of several types of psychosis (Brodie et al., 1959; Carlsson & Kindqvist, 1963). Furthermore, in the treatment of schizophrenia, the more potent major tranquilizers have been shown to produce a higher serum level of methoxylated metabolites of dopamine (Carlsson & Lind qvist, 1963). This factor tends to substantiate the theory of dopamine inhibition. Inhibition yields a higher concentration of dopamine in the synapse, rendering more of it available for synaptic destruction to inactive metabolites.

Four theories place mechanisms of action at the structure or organ/ system level. Major tranquilizers are believed to decrease the amount of extraneous incoming stimuli to the cerebral cortex (Chen & Poim, 1963), presumably via the reticular activating system (Himwich & Rinald, 1957). They also are believed to act at the level of the limbic system (Lipton et al., 1978) to reduce the affective or emotional charge on incoming stimuli (Hollister, 1973). These two theories account for the therapeutic benefit of these agents. Two additional theories relate to secondary considerations in the use of major tranquilizers. One places the mechanism of action at the level of the hypothalamic-pituitary axis, where the action appears to be reduction of the peripheral physiological response to affectively charged incoming stimuli. This response reduction might possibly account for the effects of autonomic blocking seen as side effects of these agents (Anden, 1974; Anden et al., 1970). The fourth theory places the locus of action at the level of the basal ganglia. Because it is known that dopamine is reduced in the brains of individuals with parkinsonism and many other diseases of the basal ganglia, it can be understood how these agents, inhibiting dopamine as they do, can produce certain of the characteristic extrapyramidal side effects associated with major tranquilizers (Hollister, 1973; Clement-Cormier et al., 1974).

PRINCIPLES OF USE

Selection of a Component Drug

From a therapeutic standpoint, all the major tranquilizers mentioned in Table 3–1 have been found to be equally efficacious for the psychiatric states indicated (Casey & Lasky et al., 1960; Casey & Bennet et al., 1960; Adelson & Epstein, 1962; Cole, 1964; Schiele et al., 1961; Fincle & Johnson, 1965; Gallant et al., 1965; Gallant et al., 1966, Bishop et al., 1966; Samuels, 1961; Prasad & Townley, 1966; Klein & Davis, 1969). Therefore, other factors influence selection of one drug or subgroup over another. Some of these considerations include the following.

Presence of desired aspects, such as:
    1.   A soporific component, useful for a sleep disturbance that is part of a major tranquilizer-responsive syndrome.
    2.   The patient's past history of good therapeutic response to the specific drug.
    3.   Previous experience of the physician with a particular component member of the drug, as long as there is no current contraindication to the use of the specific agent.

Absence of undesirable effects, such as:
    1.   Possibility of an adverse response to the agent's soporific or sedating effects, as in paranoid patients who wish to avoid any lessening of a vigilant state. The most soporific agents are the aliphatic and piperidine subgroups in the phenothiazine group, followed in decreasing order of soporific potential by the dihydroindolones, dibenzoxazepines, thioxanthenes, the piperazine phenothiazines, and the butyrophenones.[1]
    2.   Abnormal physiological state or states potentially worsened by the predominance of (a) certain said effect(s); for example,
        a.   Anticholinergic effects in a patient with a history of urinary hesitancy or in a patient with glaucoma (see Table 3–2 for a comparison of anticholinergic potential) (DeMaio, 1972; Snyder et al., 1974).
        b.   Antidopaminergic effects in a patient with idiopathic parkinsonism (see Table 3–3 for a comparison of antidopaminergic potential) (Snyder et al., 1978).

---

[1]The relative soporific potentials of loxapine and molindone are not clear, although they seem to be more soporific than piperazine phenothiazine compounds.

Table 3–2

Relative Comparisons of Major Tranquilizers with Respect to Their Anticholinergic Potential (Numerical Values in Increasing Order of Potential)

Group or Subgroup	Anticholinergic Potential
Butyrophenone	1
Phenothiazine—Piperazines	2
Thioxanthenes	3
Dibenzoxazepines[a]	4
Dihydroindolones	4
Phenothiazine—Aliphatic	5
Phenothiazine—Piperdines	6

[a]Their exact position in the anticholinergic spectrum is inconclusive.

Table 3–3

Relative Comparisons of Major Tranquilizers with Respect to Their Antidopaminergic Potential (Numerical Values in Decreasing Order of Potential)

Group or Subgroup	Antidopaminergic Potential[a]
Butyrophenone	6
Phenothizine—Piperazines	5
Thioxanthenes	4
Dibenzoxapines[b]	3
Dihydroindolones[b]	3
Phenothiazine—Aliphatic	2
Phenothiazine—Piperdine	1

[a]Note that the antidopaminergic potential is inversely proportionate to the anticholinergic potential; that is, the more antidopaminergic an agent is, the less anticholinergic it is. This is believed to be because acetylcholine and dopamine are in inverse proportion to each other in the brain. Consequently, as dopamine is decreased, acetylcholine is increased, and more antidopaminergic agents have less anticholinergic effects. Therefore, the pharmacological approach to major-tranquilizer-induced antidopaminergic syndromes (e.g., extraphramidal effects: parkinsonism, acute dystonias and dyskinesias, as well as akathisia) should consist of treatment with an anticholinergic agent such as trihexphenidyl hydrochloride (Artane®), benztropine methanesulfonate (Cogentin®), or diphendydramine (Benadryl®). These anticholinergic agents have the potential for restoring balance to the brain acetylcholine-dopamine axis by decreasing acetylcholine, correcting the dopamine deficiency state. Tardive dyskinesia, another major-tranquilizer-induced extrapyramidal side effect, unlike the others, is believed to result from a relative predominance of dopamine. Etiological considerations of this state are mentioned in Table 3–5, in the column "side effects." Suffice it to say, however, that anticholinergic agents can either produce or worsen this syndrome in a predisposed individual. To decrease acetylcholine causes an increase in dopamine—the purported etiology of tardive dyskinesia. Existing treatment regimens for tardive dyskinesia have, in most cases, been relatively unsuccessful, but the rationale is still the need to lower the dopamine. Therefore, regimens that have been developed include such agents as deanol (Deaner®), an acetylcholine precursor, pure choline, and physostigmine (an acetylcholinesterase inhibitor that decreases the destruction of acetylcholine and increases its brain concentration).

[b]Their exact position in the antidopaminergic spectrum remains inconclusive at this time.

26

Contraindications

Absolute.
1. Previous hypersensitivity reaction (allergic).
2. Declining level of central nervous system consciousness, either from intracerebral causes (e.g., elevation of intracranial pressure) or extracerebral causes (e.g., alcohol).

Relative. If a patient's physiological homeostasis is threatened by the side effects of the drug of choice, the final decision to use a major tranquilizer must include considerations as to whether the disadvantages of disrupting homeostasis outweigh the advantages of the drug's therapeutic benefit. This is seldom the case. Furthermore, even when there are not serious relative contraindications, consultations with other appropriate specialists and close monitoring may very well be indicated.

Indications for Use in
Functional Psychiatric Disorders[2]

Any syndrome accompanied by incipient or manifest delusions, hallucinations, or incipient or manifest schizophrenia. For example, for a patient presenting with depression accompanied by one of these states, the initial psychotropic choice is a major tranquilizer. This same class would also constitute the initial psychopharmacologic agents were hypomania or mania associated with one of these states (see Chapter 6 for elaboration).

Anxious depression or anxiety of moderate to severe intensity (Overall et al., 1966; Fink et al., 1965) accompanied by one or more of the states noted in the last paragraph, requires major tranquilizers. However, the indicated treatment for anxiety or anxious depression alone is based on intensity. Specifically, anxiety or anxious depression of moderate to severe intensity requires major tranquilizers. Minor tranquilizers are indicated for mild severity of these two states (see Chapter 4 for elaboration).

Agitation accompanying acute mania or hypomania necessitates major tranquilizers for the agitation, with lithium carbonate for the hypomania and mania.

Hypomania or mania accompanied by incipient delusions, manifest delu-

---

[2]It should be restated that if thorough evaluation of any one of the clinical states in this section suggests a presumed or apparent organic origin, the clinical approach is to identify and reverse it. If such an origin does not exist, or cannot be reversed, the same indications for major tranquilizers exist as with functional disorders, assuming no absolute or significant relativ contraindications exist. Physician evaluation and judgment must provide the basis for such decisions.

sions, or hallucinations is also treated with a combined regimen of major tranquilizers or lithium.

Hypomania or mania accompanied by incipient or manifest schizophrenia is treated with major tranquilizers alone (see Chapter 7 for elaboration).

Dosage Regimens

The essential components of a dosage regimen include starting dosage, incremental stages enroute to the production of remission, plateau dosage (the lowest dosage required to produce remission of the acute state), decremental stages to the maintenance dosage level, and the maintenance dosage level itself (the lowest dosage required to maintain remission). Key factors affecting dosage regimens are the following.

Age.   Generally speaking, persons younger than 18 or older than 55–60 should receive approximately one-fourth to one-third the normal dosage. These are arbitrary age limits, but should be considered as guidelines. Before age 18 metabolic functioning may be immature; beyond 55–60 there is a reduction in metabolic integrity.

Stature.   Patients of slight or frail stature should ideally receive one-fourth to one-third the normal dosage. On the other hand, obese persons should not receive increased dosage.

Equivalence.   Two types of equivalence should be considered in the determination of dosage regimens.

1.   Intramuscularly (I.M.) versus per os (orally) (P.O.) administered. Intramuscularly administered major tranquilizers are approximately 3–4 times more potent than the same dose given orally. For example, chlorpromazine (Thorazine) 25 mg. I.M. is approximately equivalent in potency to 75–100 mg. P.O. (Hollister, 1973).

2.   Relative equipotence of the major tranquilizers. Table 3–4 shows approximately equivalent dosages (Davis, 1974). For example, if chlorpromazine administered at 200 mg. per day would constitute an acceptable starting dosage, thiothixine (Navane®), being 25 times more potent, would be described at 8 mg. per day.

Disease state.   The various psychiatric diagnostic entities described under "Indications for Use in Functional Psychiatric Disorders," above, may require different starting, incremental, plateau, decremental, and maintenance dosages. These are generally administered orally in tablet, capsule, or concentrate forms, but relatively recent research has demonstrated the intramuscular route to be potentially effective in the production of remission from the acute illness (Goldstein & Clyde, 1966; Lafave, 1967).

Table 3–4.
Comparison of Potencies between Major Tranquilizers (Administered Orally)

Groups	Relative Equipotencies
Phenothiazines	
Aliphatic subgroup	
chlorpromazine (Thorazine, CPZ)	1
Piperidine subgroup	
thioridazine (Mellaril®)	1
mesoridazine (Serentil®)	2/3
Piperazine subgroup	
acetophenazine (Tindal®)	1/5
prochlorperazine (Compazine®)	1/6
perphenazine (Trilafon®)	1/10
trifluoperazine (Stelazine®)	1/20
fluphenazine (Prolixin®)	1/50
Thioxanthenes	
thiothixene (Navane®)	1/25
chlorprothixene (Taractan®)	1
Butyrophenone	
haloperidol (Haldol®)	1/50
Dibenzoxazepine	
loxapine succinate (Loxitane®)	1/10
Dihydroindolone	
molindone (Moban®)	1/10

The goal of major tranquilizer treatment is remission of the acute state, whether it is a first occurrence or an exacerbation of a chronic condition. This is a key concept. These agents are used too often purely as a means of chemical control of symptoms and signs. However, the major tranquilizers have not necessarily been demonstrated to eradicate the underlying origin of psychiatric illness.

Before a discussion of suggested major tranquilizer regimens for the indicated psychiatric state, three points should be mentioned. First, these regimens have been found to be extremely effective. Second, the dosage regimens presented do not account for age, stature, or equivalence. Therefore, appropriate dosage corrections will have to be made to suit the requirements of each patient. Third, the regimens presented here treat chlorpromazine as the model because it has an assigned potency value of 1. If another major tranquilizer is selected, further dosage corrections will have to be made.

1. For psychiatric states including incipient or manifest schizophrenia, incipient or manifest delusions, and/or hallucinations, the starting

dose of chlorpromazine is 200–300 mg. per day, either in once-a-day or divided daily dosage. The dosage is increased by 100 mg. every or every other day until remission is obtained, or until *significant* side effects ensue. The patient remains on the lowest dosage required to produce remission for approximately one month. At the end of the month, assuming remission continues, the dosage is gradually decreased by approximately one-fifth to one-sixth every several days until the maintenance level is reached. This generally is approximately one-third to one-fourth of the dosage required to produce remission. Unless absolutely indicated, major tranquilizers should never be withdrawn abruptly, because a withdrawal reaction may occur (Brooks, 1959; Judah et al., 1961; Simpson et al., 1965).

For those states that include only incipient schizophrenia, incipient or manifest delusions, and/or hallucinations, the patient should be given maintenance dosage for approximately one year. If these states recur after medication is stopped, a continuing maintenance regimen should be considered.

For *first-occurrence* acute schizophrenia, no definite length of maintenance treatment has been established. Some researchers and clinicians feel that with remission the patient gradually may be withdrawn from the major tranquilizers. Others suggest that maintenance should continue for approximately one year; yet others argue that lifetime maintenance with major tranquilizers is indicated. It seems imprudent to discontinue the agent at remission and reasonable to prescribe it for at least one year. Most researchers and clinicians agree, however, that more than one occurrence of acute schizophrenia requires continuing lifetime treatment with major tranquilizers because these agents have been shown to reduce considerably the recurrence of this potentially devastating illness (Caffey et al., 1964; Gantz and Birkett, 1965).

2. For anxious depressions or anxiety of moderate to severe intensity, the starting dosage is usually lower than for the above-mentioned states. Chlorpromazine 50–100 mg. (in once-a-day or divided dosage) is usually sufficient. The dosage is increased by 25–50 mg. every day or every other day until remission, or until significant side effects occur. The patient is maintained at that dosage level for approximately one month. At this time the dosage gradually may be reduced by approximately one-fifth to one-sixth every several days, to the lowest dosage required to maintain remission (usually one-third to one-fourth the dosage required to produce remission). The patient is maintained on the agent for approximately six months. Abrupt discontinuation of major tranquilizers may result in withdrawal effects.

3. For the agitation accompanying acute hypomania or mania, the starting dosage of chlorpromazine usually varies between 50 mg. and 200 mg. per day (in once-a-day or divided dosages), in association with lithium.

The increments from that point may be from 25 mg. to approximately 100 mg. every day or every other day until remission of this agitation. After the six to 10 days usually required to attain sufficient tissue levels of the lithium, and assuming that the agitation has considerably lessened or has abated, the clinician may wish to begin a trial gradual decrease of the major tranquilizer. Because lithium is the agent of choice for pure acute mania or hypomania, continued administration of a major tranquilizer may confuse the issue of which agent is ameliorating the agitation.

As regards the parenteral administration of major tranquilizers, three types of clinical use are generally appropriate.

1.   These agents are used for the emergency control of acute agitation that is part of a major-tranquilizer-responsive state. Usually the more sedation-producing agents, such as chlorpromazine (Thorazine, CPZ), mesoridazine (Serentil®), or haloperidol (Haldol®) are prescribed. An order should ideally be written for the specific dosage of the selected agent "every six hours p.r.n. [*pro re nata*, or 'as needed for'] unmanageable agitation." The usual intramuscular dosage of chlorpromazine is 25 mg.–50 mg. every six hours, as needed for unmanageable agitation. If an agent other than chlorpromazine is selected, its dosage must be computed on the basis of its equipotence to chlorpromazine. For example, if the I.M. dose for chlorpromazine is 50 mg., the equipotent dose for haloperidol would be 1 mg. (Haldol® is approximately 50 times more potent than chlorpromazine). Remember that any drug administered by injection is three to four times more potent than the same dosage administered orally. For example, 25 mg. of chlorpromazine I.M. is equipotent to 75–100 mg. P.O. Therefore, caution against the use of an inappropriately high intramuscular dosage must be the rule.

2.   Intramuscularly administered major tranquilizers may be used in a predetermined regimen to bring about remission. The principles of dosage regimens elaborated earlier apply to this treatment. This treatment has been found to produce rapid remission rates, and is also extremely useful for patients who will not take indicated major tranquilizers orally (Levenson, 1976; Levenson et al., 1976).

3.   Parenterally administered major tranquilizers may be effective in maintaining remission in major-tranquilizer-responsive states. The agent for this use would be fluphenazine in the decanoate form (Prolixin® decanoate), an ester compound. Once injected into the muscle mass, the ester bond is believed to be hydrolyzed by the muscle esterases, with a release of fluphenazine into the bloodstream in a timed-release fashion. Fluphenazine decanoate is especially helpful for patients who have complied poorly with prescribed psychotropic medication regimens intended

to prevent deterioration of the clinical condition. The usual dosage of this compound is 25 mg. I.M. every one to three weeks. However, there are three major considerations in selecting this agent. First, a careful assess- ment of the possible reasons for noncompliance with the use of psychotro- pic agents should be made before establishing a prognosis and indicating a therapeutic format change. Second, it is wise to consider dosage equiva- lence guidelines before prescribing fluphenazine decanoate for mainte- nance. For example, if a patient has been on an oral regimen of major tranquilizers, the appropriate bioequivalence adjustments should precede the initiation of an intramuscular regimen. If a patient has been on an acute-illness-phase, intramuscularly administered regimen, the bioe- quivalence problem would be less complex. Third, some researchers and clinicians have advocated the use of fluphenazine decanoate for acute major-tranquilizer-responsive states. Although this use may have some history of effectiveness, it precludes a carefully conceived daily or every- other-day titration regimen to remission, as in parenteral quick-acting or oral forms, since dosages of the long-acting form tend to be fixed.

Assessment

It should be underscored that, regardless of the regimen or disease state, psychiatric assessment for disposition on psychopharmacotherapy (see Chapter 7) must precede not only major tranquilizer prescription but *every* change in dosage regimen as well. The agents should never be started, nor should dosages be changed for therapeutic reasons, until there is concrete justification. This implies frequent assessment (daily or every other day) until remission is obtained. Assessment may become somewhat less fre- quent during gradation downward to maintenance levels. Any patient on major tranquilizer maintenance, however, should be evaluated at least monthly, or more often as indicated.

SIDE EFFECTS

Table 3–5 lists the majority of reported side effects of major tranquilizers and some of their purported mechanisms of production, as well as com- monly implicated groups or agents. It should be emphasized that delineat- ing these side effects is intended not to alarm the clinician but to stress the considerations in prescribing major tranquilizers. These are not innocuous agents. Therefore, they should be prescribed, and their dosage increased, only when indicated by psychiatric assessment and not contraindicated by physiological assessment. Knowledge of side effects provides the practitioner with a firmer base by which to monitor the patient's clinical course. Familiarity with side effects, regardless of how rare their occurrence, provides additional input when considering relative contraindications to prescription and continuation of these agents. A basic work-up is essential before prescription. In addition to the history, medical review of symptoms by system (MROSS), past medical history (PHMx), and physical examination, laboratory determinations are necessary, including:

- c.b.c. (complete blood count) with differential,
- serum electrolytes,
- BUN (blood urea nitrogen),
- creatinine,
- SGOT (serum glutamic-oxaloacetic transaminase),
- SGPT (serum glutamic-pyruvic transaminase),
- total and direct bilirubin,
- alkaline phosphatase,
- T_3/T_4 (triiodothyronine/thyroxine),
- routine urinalysis,
- chest x-ray,
- EKG (electrocardiogram).

Naturally, if there are any questions as to the advisability of major tranquilizer prescription, the appropriate additional laboratory studies and consultations with other specialists should be obtained. A definite protocol for laboratory reevaluation during the course of major tranquilizer treatment has not been determined, but it is recommended that the abovementioned tests be collected at least every six months. These specific tests or others may be needed sooner if there are physiological indications.

Table 3–5 follows on pages 34 through 39.

Table 3-5
Side Effects of Major Tranquilizers

Side Effects	Purported Mechanism of Production	Commonly Implicated Groups or Agents
I. Vital Signs		
A. *Blood pressure.* Orthostatic hypotension (hypotension resulting from change from lying to sitting or standing or sitting to standing positions) in most cases; severe cases have hypotension in supine (lying flat on back) position (Klein & Davis, 1969; Hollister, 1973)	Anticholinergic and/or alpha blocking	The more anticholinergic agents
B. *Pulse rate.* Tachycardia (increased heart rate)	Compensatory in response to hypotension (reduction in blood pressure reduces blood flow to tissues, requiring more rapid heart rate to pump more blood per unit of time to compensate	Same
C. *Respiratory rate.* Tachypnea (increased breathing) (Plachta, 1965)	Depressed bronchociliary action producing formation of mucus plug(s), which may cause respiratory compromise and consequent tachypnea	Chlorpromazine, but all have the potential
D. *Temperature* (see XII, B)		
E. *Weight.* Increase (Singh et al., 1970; Klett & Caffey, 1960)	Possibly mediated via action on the hypothalamic appetite centers	Aliphatic and piperidine phenothiazines
II. Central Nervous System		
A. *Sedation.* Usually self-limited, ending approximately two to three weeks after final increase of medication (Hollister, 1964)	Possibly secondary to depression of reticular activating system	The more anticholinergic agents, but all have the potential

B. *Organic brain syndrome* (Lipton et al., 1978; DiMascio & Demirgian, 1970; Haefner et al., 1965)	Depression of cerebrocortical neuronal metabolism or an anticholinergic mechanism are two possibilities	All have the potential
C. *Worsening of psychosis* (El-Yousef et al., 1973)	As acetylcholine decreases, dopamine increases in brain; elevated dopamine implicated in production of certain psychoses	All have the potential, but risk increases with more anticholinergic agents
D. *Lowering of seizure threshold* (Wittenborn et al., 1969; Maynert et al., 1975)	Mechanism unknown	Chlorpromazine, but all have the potential; tends to occur with excessively high starting or incremental dosages
E. *Extrapyramidal disorders* (Denny-Brown, 1962; Hornykiewicz, 1972; Marsden et al., 1975; Meltzer & Stahl, 1976)		
1. *Parkinsonism.* Hypokinesia, masklike faces, drooling, stooped posture, loss of associated arm movements on walking, shuffling gait, cogwheel rigidity: usually has its onset 5–20 days after onset of major tranquilizer treatment	Dopamine decrease at level of basal ganglia, produced by dopamine inhibition	The more antidopaminergic agents, although all have the potential
2. *Acute dystonia and dyskinesia.*	Dopamine decrease at level of basal ganglia, produced by dopamine inhibition	The more antidopaminergic agents, although all have the potential
a. *Dystonia.* Irregular, nonrhythmical, involuntary movements or postures of the trunk, limbs, face, tongue or neck; including retrocollis (fixed posterior movement of head), tortocollis (fixed lateral movement of head), opisthotonus (fixed arching of the back), and oculogyric crisis (head and eyes turned superiorly): usually has its onset one hour to five days after onset of major tranquilizer treatment		

Table 3-5 (continued)
Side Effects of Major Tranquilizers

Side Effects	Purported Mechanism of Production	Commonly Implicated Groups or Agents
b. *Dyskinesia.* Rhythmical, involuntary movements of the trunk and limbs: usually has its onset one hour to five days after onset of major tranquilizer treatment	Dopamine decrease at level of basal ganglia produced by dopamine inhibition	The more antidopaminergic agents, although all have the potential
3. *Akathisia.* Motor restlessness; the individual cannot sit still for longer than a few seconds: onset usually five to 40 days from onset of major tranquilizer treatment		
4. *Tardive dyskinesia.* Lip smacking, darting tongue (like a frog catching flies), inconsistent lateral jaw movements, all of which may be accompanied by axial hyperkinesis (anterior-posterior rocking of trunk), tonic contractions of neck, choreoathetoid movements of fingers and toes, and foot tapping: onset usually after 100 days of major tranquilizer therapy	Dopamine increase at level of basal ganglia, exact mechanism of production unknown; however, two theories of dopamine excess: **a)** lowering of acetylcholine, which produces relative elevation of dopamine **b)** prolonged dopamine inhibition with increased dopamine excretion from presynaptic neuron, via a positive feedback	May be produced by chronic major tranquilizer therapy, or by the addition of a more anticholinergic major tranquilizer or another agent with anticholinergic properties in predisposed individuals
III. Eyes		
A. *Retina.* Retinitis pigmentosa-like syndrome (Klein & Davis, 1969)	Mechanism unknown	Thioridazine in dosages of greater than 800 mg. per day
B. *Anterior compartment.*		
1. *Anterior lens and posterior cornea.* Deposition of pigment (Barnes & Cameron, 1966; Barsa et al., 1965; Delong et al., 1965)	Mechanism unknown	Long-term, high-dose chlorpromazine

36

2. *Blurring of vision and potential intraocular pressure increase* (Koelle, 1975)	Anticholinergic-induced mydriasis, producing decreased accommodation and impingement on the canal of Schlemm, impeding egress of intraocular fluid from the anterior chamber of the eye	Although all have the potential, risk is higher with the more anticholinergic agents
IV. Nose		
Dryness, stuffiness	Anticholinergic-induced drying of mucous membrane secretions	The more anticholinergic agents, although all have the potential
V. Mouth		
A. *Dryness with occasional thirst* (Van der Kolk et al., 1978)	Same as for the nose	Same
B. *Few reported cases of oral moniliasis* (Kane, 1963a and b; Kane & Anderson, 1964)	Oral moniliasis may occur when sugar-containing substances are consumed	Same
VI. Neck		
Increased PBI and I_{131} uptake	Mechanism unknown	Perphenazine and chlorpromazine; however, inconclusive
VII. Thorax		
A. *Bronchopulmonary axis.* Tachypnea	See I, C	See I, C
B. *Heart.* Prolonged Q-R interval and depressed or inverted T-wave on EKG, ventricular arrhythmias (Wendkos, 1964; Leestma & Koenig, 1968; Lutz, 1976; Fowler et al., 1976; Alvared-Mena & Frank, 1973; Ayd, 1972; Baldessarini, 1977)	Mechanism unknown; however, believed to be benign repolarization effects, in part	The more anticholinergic agents, although all have the potential
C. *Breasts (female).* Galactorrhea (Sachar, 1978)	Mechanism unknown; however, possibly results from action of agents on hypothalamic-pituitary axis	Piperidine and aliphatic phenothiazines

Table 3–5 (continued)
Side Effects of Major Tranquilizers

Side Effects	Purported Mechanism of Production	Commonly Implicated Groups or Agents
VIII. Abdomen		
A. *Gastrointestinal tract.* Constipation, dysphagia (Ayd, 1960; Greenblatt et al., 1964; Hollister et al., 1960; Efron, 1968; Waldrop et al., 1961; Hussar & Bragg, 1969)	Anticholinergic-induced hypoperistalsis	The more anticholinergic agents, although all have the potential
B. *Liver.* Various degrees of an acute hepatitis-like syndrome, including malaise, lassitude, nausea, vomiting, abdominal pain, hepatomegaly, jaundice, pruritis, and abnormalities in one or more liver-function tests (SGOT, SGPT, total/direct bilirubin, alkaline phosphatase) (Klein & Davis, 1969; Barancik, et al., 1967; Hollister, 1958, 1959)	An allergic hypersensitivity-induced accumulation of eosinophils within small bile ducts of liver, producing a cholestatic obstruction	Chlorpromazine, although all except loxapine succinate have the potential
IX. Reproductive Tract		
A. *Female.* Hypomenorrhea or amenorrhea (Klein & Davis, 1969)	Exact mechanism unknown, but possibly result of action of agents on hypothalamic-pituitary axis; confusion exists about whether this or emotionality or both are responsible for his menstrual problem	Chlorpromazine and thioridazine
B. *Male.* Impotence, inhibition of ejaculation, retrograde ejaculation (Brill, 1958; Freyhan, 1961; Shader, 1972; Greenberg, 1971; Ditman, 1964)	Presumably due to anticholinergic and/or sympatholytic effect	The more anticholinergic agents, especially thioridazine
X. Urinary Tract Function		
Urinary hesitancy and retention (Merrill & Markland, 1970; Merrill & Markland, 1972)	Presumably secondary to anticholinergic effect	The more anticholinergic agents, although all have the potential

XI. Skin

(Klein & Davis, 1969; Ban & Lehmann, 1965; Ban et al., 1965; Feldman & Frierson, 1964; Greiner et al., 1964)

A. *Diffuse maculopapular urticaria.*	Systemic hypersensitivity reaction; local hypersensitivity from contact of agent and skin; deposition of pigment subepidermally, precipitated by exposure to sun	All have the potential
B. *Localized contact dermatitis-like picture.*		
C. *Photosensitivity reaction,* Sun-exposed areas demonstrate sunburn-like picture, which, without treatment, may progress to brown to purplish to bluish areas of pigmentation ("slate-blue skin")		Chlorpromazine Long-term, high-dose chlorpromazine

XII. Hematopoietic System

(Anglejan et al., 1965; Pretty et al., 1965; Reznikoff, 1961; Rosenthal et al., 1967)

A. *Pancytopenia.*	Bone marrow suppression; direct toxicity suspected; however, exact mechanism unknown	Fluphenazine, but all have potential
B. *Agranulocytosis.* Manifested by elevated temperature and sore throat; pharyngeal inspection usually reveals erythema and ulcerations, and the c.b.c. shows a decline and/or significant reduction to only a few white cells, specifically neutrophils; may occur at any time after major tranquilizer treatment initiation, but is usually seen between six and eleventh week of therapy; any evidence of sore throat and/or elevated temperature requires immediate c.b.c. with differential and serial c.b.c.s with differential, as indicated, regardless of the duration of major tranquilizer treatment		Chlorpromazine, but all have potential

40 Basic Psychopharmacology

REFERENCES

Adelson, D., and Epstein, L. J. A Study of Phenothiazines with Male and Female Chronically Ill Schizophrenic Patients. *J. Nerv. Ment. Dis.*, 1962, 134:543.

Alvared-Mena, S. C., and Frank, J. J. Phenothiazine Induced T-Wave Abnormalities. *JAMA*, 1973, 224:1730.

Anden, N.-E. The Interaction of Neuroleptic Drugs with Striatal and Limbic Dopaminergic Mechanisms, in G. Sedvall, B. Unvas, and Y. Zotterman (eds.), *Antipsychotic Drugs: Pharmacodynamics and Pharmacokinetics*. Pergamon Press, Oxford, 1974, pp. 217–225.

Anden, N.-E., Butcher, S. G., Corrodi, H., Fuxe, K., and Understedt, V. Receptor Activity and Turnover of Dopamine and Noradrenaline after Neurolep tics. *Eur. J. Pharmacol.*, 1970, 11:303.

Anglejan, G., Dausset, J., and Bernard, J. Blood Disorders Induced by Phenothiazines. *Bull. Soc. Med. Hosp.*, 1965, 116:507.

Ayd, F. J. Haloperidol: Fifteen Years of Clinical Experience. *Dis. Nerv. Syst.*, 1972, 33:459.

———. Amitriptyline (Elavil) Therapy for Depressive Reactions. *Psychomatics*, 1960, 1:320.

Baldessarini, R. J. *Chemotherapy in Psychiatry*. Harvard University Press, Cambridge, Mass., 1977.

Ban, T. A., and Lehmann, H. E., Skin Pigmentation, a Rare Side Effect of Chlorpromazine. *Canad. Psychiat. Assn. J.*, 1965, 10:112.

Ban, T. A., Lehmann, H. E., Gallai, Z., Warnes, H., and Lee, H. Relationship between Photosensitivity and Pathological Pigmentation of Chlorpromazine. *Union. Med. Canada.*, 1965, 94:305.

Barancik, M., Brandenborg, L. L., and Albion, M. J. Thioridazine-Induced Cholestasis. *JAMA*, 1967, 200:69.

Barnes, G. J., and Cameron, M. D. Skin and Eye Changes Associated with Chlorpromazine Therapy. *Med. J. Aust.*, 1966, 1:478.

Barsa, J. A., Newton, J. C., and Saunders, J. C. Lenticular and Corneal Opacities during Phenothiazine Therapy. *JAMA*, 1965, 193:10.

Bishop, M. P., Fulmer, T. E., and Gallant, D. M. Thiothixene versus Trifluoperazine in Newly Admitted Schizophrenic Patients. *Curr. Ther. Res.*, 1966, 8:509.

Brill, V. A. (ed.). *Pharmacology in Medicine* (2nd ed.). McGraw-Hill, New York, 1958.

Brodie, B. B., Spector, S., and Shore, P. A. Interaction Drugs with Norepinephrine in the Brain. *Pharmacol. Rev.*, 1959, 11:548.

Brooks, G. W.: Withdrawal from Neuroleptic Drugs. *Amer. J. Psychiat.*, 1959, 115:93.

Burt, D. R., Creese, I., and Snyder, S. H. Properties of [3H] Haloperidol and [3H] Dopamine Binding Associated with Dopamine Receptors in Calf Brain Membranes. *Mol. Pharmacol.*, 1976, 12:800.

Caffey, E. M., Diamond, L. S., Frank, T. V., Grasberger, J. C., Herman, L.,

Klett, C. J., and Rothstein, C. Discontinuation on Reduction of Chemotherapy in Chronic Schizophrenics. *J. Chronic. Dis.*, 1964, *17*:347.

Carlsson, A., and Lindquist, M. Effect of Chlorpromazine Haloperidol on Formation of 3-Methoxytyramine and Normetanephrine in Mouse Brain. *Acta. Pharmacol. Et Toxicol.*, 1963, *20*:140.

Casey, J. F., Bennett, I. R., Lindley, C. J., Hollister, L. E., Gordon, M. H., and Springer, N. N. Drug Therapy in Schizophrenia. A Controlled Study of the Relative Effectiveness of Chlorpromazine, Promazine, Phenobarbital, and Placebo. *Arch. Gen. Psychiat.* 1960, *2*:210.

Casey, J. F., Lasky, J. J., Klett, C. J., and Hollister, L. E. Treatment of Schizophrenic Reactions with Phenothiazine Derivatives. A Comparative Study of Chlorpromazine, Trifluopromazine, Mepazine, Prochlorperazine, Perphenazine, and Phenobarbital. *Am. J. Psychiat.*, 1960, *117*:97.

Chen, C. H., and Poim, S. Carphenazine in the Treatment of Schizophrenia. *Curr. Ther. Res.*, 1963, *5*:195.

Clement-Cormier, Y. C., Kebabian, J. W., Petzold, G. L., and Greengard, P. Dopamine-Sensitive Adenylate Cyclase in Mammalian Brain: A Possible Site of Action of Antipsychotic Drugs. *Proc. Nat. Acad. Sci. USA*, 1974, *71*:1113.

Cole, J. D. Phenothiazine Treatment in Acute Schizophrenia. *Arch. Gen. Psychiat.*, 1964, *10*:246.

Davis, J. M. Dose Equivalence of the Antipsychotic Drugs. *J. Psychiat. Res.*, 1974, *11*:65.

Delong, S. L., Poley, B. J., and McFarlane, J. R., Jr., Ocular Changes Associated with Long-term Chlorpromazine Therapy. *Arch. Opthal.*, 1965, *73*:611.

DeMaio, D. Clozapine, a Novel Major Tranquilizer: Clinical Experiences and Pharmacotherapeutic Hypotheses. *Arzneim-Forsch*, 1972, *22*:919.

Denny-Brown, D. *The Basal Ganglia and Their Relations to Disorders of Movement.* Oxford University Press, London, 1962.

DiMascio, A., and Demirgian, E. Antiparkinson Drug Overuse. *Psychosomatics*, 1970, *11*:596.

Ditman, K. S. Comparative Chemotherapeutic Trial in Treatment of Chronic Borderline Patients. *Am. J. Psychiat.* 1964, *120*:1004.

Efron, D. *Psychopharmacology: A Review Of Progress, 1957–1967.* U.S. Government Printing Office, Washington, D.C., 1968.

El-Yousef, M. K., Janowsky, D. S., Davis, J. M., and Sekerke, H. J. Reversal of Antiparkinsonian Drug Toxicity by Physostigmine: A Controlled Study. *Am. J. Psychiat.*, 1973, *130*:141.

Fann, W. E., Davis, J. M., Janowsky, D. S., Sekerke, H. J., and Schmidt, D. M. Chlorpromazine: Effects of Antacids on Its Gastrointestinal Absorption. *J. Clin. Pharmacol.*, 1973, *10*:388.

Feldman, P. E., and Frierson, B. D. Dermatological and Opthamological Changes Associated with Prolonged Chlorpromazine Therapy. *Am. J. Psychiat.*, 1964, *121*:187.

Fincle, L. P., and Johnson, C. C. Psychiatric and Behavioral Effects of Chlorprothixene Concentrate Suspension in Chronic Hospitalized Schizophrenics. *Dis. Nerv. Syst.*, 1965, *26*:225.

42 Basic Psychopharmacology

Fink, M., Klein, D. F., and Kramer, J. C. Clinical Efficacy of Chlorpromazine Procyclidine Combination, Imipramine and Placebo in Depressive Disorders. *Psychopharmacologia*, 1965, 7:27.

Forrest, I. S., Bolt, A. G., and Serra, M. T. Distribution of Chlorpromazine Metabolites in Selected Organs of Psychiatric Patients Chronically Dosed up to the Time of Death. *Biochem. Pharmacol.*, 1968, 17:2061.

Fowler, N. D., McCall, D., Chou, T.-C., Holmes, S. C., and Hanenson, I. B. Electrocardiographic Changes and Cardiac Arrhythmias in Patients Receiving Psychotropic Drugs. *Am. J. Cardiol.*, 1976, 37:223.

Freyhan, F. A. Loss of Ejaculation During Mellaril Treatment. *Am. J. Psychiat.*, 1961, 118:171.

Gallant, D. M., Bishop, M. P., and Sprehe, D. A New Thioridazine Derivative. *Curr. Ther. Res.*, 1965, 7:102.

Gallant, D. M., Bishop, M. P., Timmons, E., and Gould, A. R. Thiothixene (P4657B): Controlled Evaluation in Chronic Schizophrenic Patients. *Curr. Ther. Res.*, 1966, 8:153.

Gantz, R. S., and Birkett, D. P. Phenothiazine Reduction as a Cause of Rehospitalization. *Arch. Gen. Psychiatr.*, 1965, 12:586.

Goldstein, B. J., and Clyde, D. J. Haloperidol in Controlling the Symptoms of Acute Psychoses. II. A Double-blind Evaluation of Haloperidol and Trifluoperazine. *Curr. Ther. Res.*, 1966, 8:236.

Greenberg, H. R. Inhibition of Ejaculation by Chlorpromazine. *J. Nerv. Ment. Dis.*, 1971, 152:364.

Greenblatt, M., Grosser, G. H., and Wechsler, H. Differential Response of Hospitalized Depressed Patients to Somatic Therapy. *Am. J. Psychiat.*, 1964, 120:935.

Greiner, A. C., Nicolson, G. A., and Baker, R. A. Therapy of Chlorpromazine Melanosis: A Preliminary Report. *Canad. Med. Assn. J.*, 1964, 91:636.

Groves, J., and Mandell, M. The Long-Acting Phenothiazines. *Arch. Gen. Psychiat.*, 1975, 32:893.

Haefner, H., Heyder, B., and Kutscher, I. Undesirable Side Effects and Complications with the Use of Neuroleptic Drugs. *Int. J. Neuropsychiatry*, 1965, 1:46.

Himwich, H. E. and Rinald, F. The effect of drugs on the reticular system, in W. S. Field, *Brain Mechanisms and Drug Action*, Charles C Thomas, Springfield, Ill., 1957, pp. 15–44.

Hollister, L. E. *Clinical Use of Psychotherapeutic Drugs*, Charles C Thomas, Springfield, Ill., 1973.

———. Complications from Psychotherapeutic Drugs. *Clin. Pharmacol. Ther.*, 1964, 5:322.

———. Chlorpromazine Jaundice. JAMA, 1959, 169:1235.

———. Allergic Reactions to Tranquilizing Drugs. *Ann. Intern. Med.*, 1958, 49:17.

Hollister, L. E., Caffey, E. M., and Klett, C. H. Abnormal Symptoms, Signs, and Laboratory Tests during Treatment with Phenothiazine Derivatives. *Clin. Pharmacol. Ther.*, 1960, 1:284.

Hollister, L. E., Curry, S. H., Derr, J. E., and Kanter, S. L. Studies of Delayed-Action Medication. V. Plasma Levels and Urinary Excretion of Chlorpromazine in Four Different Dosage Forms Given Acutely and in Steadystate Conditions. *Clin. Pharmacol. Ther.*, 1970, *11*:49.

Horn, A. S., and Snyder, S. H. Chlorpromazine and Dopamine: Conformational Similarities that Correlate with the Antischizophrenic Activity of Phenothiazine Drugs. *Proc. Nat. Sci. USA.*, 1971, *68*:2325.

Hornykiewicz, O. Dopamine and Extrapyramidal Motor Function and Dysfunction, in I. J. Kopin (ed.), *Neurotransmitters*. Williams and Wilkins, Baltimore, 1972, pp. 390–415.

Hussar, A. E., and Bragg, D. G. The Effect of Chlorpromazine on the Swallowing Function in Chronic Schizophrenic Patients. *Am. J. Psychiat.*, 1969, *126*:570.

Judah, L. N., Josephs, Z. M., and Murphree, O. D. Results of Simultaneous Abrupt Withdrawal of Ataraxics in 500 Chronic Psychotic Patients. *Am. J. Psychiat.*, 1961, *118*:156.

Kane, F. J., Jr. Oral Moniliasis following the Use of Thorazine, *Am. J. Psychiat.* 1963a, *119*:890.

———. Oral Moniliasis following the Use of Thorazine. *Am. J. Psychiat.* 1963b, *120*:187.

Kane, F. J., Jr., and Anderson, W. B. A Fourth Occurrence of Oral Moniliasis during Tranquilizer Therapy. *Am. J. Psychiat.*, 1964, *120*:1199.

Klein, D. F., and Davis, J. M. *Diagnosis and Drug Treatment of Psychiatric Disorders*. Williams and Wilkins, Baltimore, 1969.

Klett, C. J., and Caffey, E. M., Jr. Weight Changes during Treatment with Phenothiazine Derivatives. *J. Neuropsychiatr.*, 1960, *2*:102.

Koelle, G. B. Neurohumoral Transmission and the Autonomic Nervous System, in L. S. Goodman and A. Gilman (eds.), *The Pharmacological Basis of Therapeutics*. Macmillan, New York, 1975, pp. 404–444.

Lafave, H. G. Haloperidol. New Addition to the Drug Treatment of Schizophrenia. *Canad. Psychiat. Assn. J.*, 1967, *12*:597.

Leestma, J. E., and Koenig, K. L. Sudden Death and Phenothiazines, *Arch. Gen. Psychiatr.*, 1968, *18*:137.

Levenson, A. J. Intramuscularly Administered Fluphenazine HCL in Acute Schizophrenia: A Retrospective Study. *Curr. Ther. Res.*, 1976, *19*:320.

Levenson, A. J., Burnett, G. B., Nottingham, J. D., Sermas, C. I., and Thornby, J. I. Speed and Rate of Remission in Acute Schizophrenia: A Comparison of Intramuscularly Administered Fluphenazine HCL with Thiothixene and Haloperidol. *Curr. Ther. Res.*, 1976, *20*:695.

Lipton, M. A., DiMascio, A., and Killam, K. F. (eds.), *Psychopharmacology: A Generation of Progress*. Raven Press, New York, 1978.

Lutz, E. G. Cardiotoxic Effects of Psychotropic Drugs. *J. Med. Soc. New Jersey*, 1976, *73*:105.

Marsden, C. D., Tarsy, D., and Baldessarini, R. J. Spontaneous and Drug-Induced Movement Disorders in Psychotic Patients, in D. F. Benson and D. Blumer (eds.), *Psychiatric Aspects of Neurologic Disease*. Grune and Stratton, New York, 1975, pp. 219–266.

Maynert, E. W., Marczynski, T. J., and Browning, R. A. The Role of The Neuro-

Transmitters in the Epilepsies, in W. S. Friedlander (ed.), *Advances in Neurology*. Vol. 13. Raven Press, New York, 1975, pp. 79–146.

McGeer, P. L. The Chemistry of Mind. *American Scientist*, 1971, 59:221.

Mednick, S. A. A Learning Theory Approach to Research in Schizophrenia. *Psychol. Bull.*, 1958, 55:315.

Meehl, P. E. Schizotoxia, Schizotypy, Schizophrenia. *Am. Psychol.*, 1962, 17:827.

Meltzer, H. Y., and Stahl, S. M. The Dopamine Hypothesis of Schizophrenia: A Review. *Schizo. Bull.*, 1976, 2:19.

Merrill, D. C., and Markland, C. A Laboratory Investigation of the Effect of Phenothiazines on Urinary Bladder Function. *Invest. Urol.*, 1970, 7:532.

———. Vesical Dysfunction Induced by the Major Tranquilizers. *J. Urol.*, 1972, 107:769.

Moyano, C. Z. A Double Blind Comparison of Loxapine Succinate and Trifluoperazine Hydrochloride in Chronic Schizophrenic Patients. *Dis. Nerv. Syst.*, 1975, 36:301.

Overall, J. E., Hollister, L. E., Johnson, M., and Pennington, V. Nosology of Depression and Differential Response to Drugs. *JAMA*, 1966, 195:946.

Plachta, A. Asphyxia Relatively Inherent to Tranquilization. *Arch. Gen. Psychiat.*, 1965, 12:152.

Prasad, L., and Townley, M. C. Haloperidol and Thioridazine in Treatment of Chronic Schizophrenics. *Dis. Nerv. Syst.*, 1966, 27:722.

Pretty, H. M., Gosselin, G., Colpron, G., and Long, L. A. Agranulocytosis: A Report of 30 Cases. *Canad. Med. Assn.*, 1965, 93:1058.

Reznikoff, L. Clinical Observations of Therapeutic Effect of Chlorprothixene in Psychoses. *Am. J. Psychiat.*, 1961, 118:348.

Rosenthal, D. S., Stein, G. F., and Santos, J. C. Thioridazine Agranulocytosis. *JAMA*, 1967, 200:81.

Sachar, E. J. Neuroendocrine Responses to Psychotropic Drugs, in M. A. Lipton, A. DiMascio, and K. F. Killam (eds.), *Psychopharmacology: A Generation of Progress*. Raven Press, New York, 1978, pp. 499–507.

Samuels, A. S. A Controlled Study of Haloperidol: The Effect of Small Dosages. *Am. J. Psychiat.*, 1961, 118:250.

Schiele, B. C., Vestre, N. D., and Stein, K. E. A Comparison of Thioridazine, Trifluoperazine, Chlorpromazine, and Placebo: A Double-Blind Controlled Study on the Treatment of Chronic, Hospitalized, Schizophrenic Patients. *J. Clin. Exp. Psychopath.*, 1961, 22:151.

Shader, R. I. Sexual Dysfunction Associated with Mesoridazine Besylate (Serentil). *Psychopharmacologia*, 1972, 27:293.

Simpson, G. M., Amin, M., and Kunz, E. Withdrawal Effects of Phenothiazines. *Compr. Psychiat.*, 1965, 6:347.

Singh, M. M., Dios, L. V., and Kline, N. S. Weight as a Clinical Correlate of Clinical Response to Psychotropic Drugs. *Psychosomatics*, 1970, 11:562.

Snyder, S. H., Banerjee, S. P., Yamamura, H. I., and Greenberg, D. Drugs, Neurotransmitters, and Schizophrenia. *Science*, 1974, 184:1243.

Snyder, S. H., U'Prichard, D. C., and Greenberg, D. A. Neurotransmitter Receptor Binding in the Brain, in M. A. Lipton, A. DiMascio, and K. F. Killam(eds.), *Psychopharmacology: A Generation of Progress*. Raven Press, New York, 1978, pp. 361–370.

Van der Kolk, B. A., Shader, R. I., and Greenblatt, D. J. Autonomic Effects of Psychotropic Drugs, in M. A. Lipton, A. DiMascio, and K. F. Killam (eds.), *Psychopharmacology: A Generation of Progress*. Raven Press, New York, 1978, pp. 1009–1020.

Waldrop, F. N., Robertson, R. H., and Vourlekis, L. A Comparison of the Therapeutic and Toxic Effects of Thioridazine and Chlorpromazine in Chronic Schizophrenic Patients. *Compr. Psychiat.*, 1961, 2:96.

Wendkos, M. H. The Significance of Electrocardiographic Changes Produced by Thioridazine. *J. New Drugs*, 1964, 4:322.

Wittenborn, J. R., Cole, J. O., and Levine, J. (eds). *Psychopharmacology: A Review of Progress, 1957–1967*. Public Health Service Publication, No. 1836, U.S. Government Printing Office, Washington, D.C., 1969.

CHAPTER 4

Minor Tranquilizers

The pharmacological groups usually considered as minor tranquilizers, and some commonly prescribed component members, are listed in Table 4–1. This chapter, however, focuses on the benzodiazepines, as they are generally in wider use and, in many cases, are potentially safer than the other minor tranquilizers. It should be underscored that despite the prevalent prescription of the benzodiazepines, much investigation needs to be done with respect to their pharmacology.

PERTINENT PHARMACOKINETICS

The benzodiazepines, administered orally, are variably absorbed through the intestinal mucosa; peak blood levels are reached in approximately one to four hours. Diazepam and lorazepam usually reach peak blood levels in approximately one to two hours.

These agents presumably cross the blood-brain barrier, although this is not known conclusively in the case of every compound. They are excreted primarily in the urine and possess varying half-lives and tissue-accumulation patterns. The half-life of oxazepam is from three to 21 hours; for lorazepam it is from three to 12 hours, respectively. These two agents are reported to have little or no tissue accumulation after steady administration. This suggests fairly rapid decreasing blood levels after discontinuation and indicates the need for split dosage regimens. On the other hand, chlordiazepoxide and diazepam have half-lives of up to approximately 96 hours, presumably partly because they produce pharmacologically active metabolites and partly because the drugs are slowly metabolized. Fur-

Table 4-1
Commonly Prescribed Minor Tranquilizers

Group	Approximate Dosage Range (in Milligrams), Either Once-a-Day or Divided Dosages as Indicated
Benzodiazepines	
diazepam (Valium®)	5–60
chlordiazepoxide hydrochloride (Librium®)	5–300
oxazepam (Serax®)	20–120
lorazepam (Ativan®)	1–6
Barbiturates	
phenobarbital	16–100
Glycerol derivatives	
meprobamate (Miltown®, Equanil®)	800–3200
tybamate	750–2000
Diphenylmethane antihistaminics	
hydroxyzine pamoate (Vistaril®)	75–400
diphenhydramine hydrochloride (Benadryl®)	25–200

thermore, these latter two agents, especially diazepam, tend to accumulate in tissues after repeated administration. Therefore, after approximately five to seven days (Greenblatt & Shader, 1974), a once-a-day dosage regimen should suffice (e.g., at bedtime in cases with an initial or intermittent sleep disturbance). Naturally, clinical conditions and the physician's judgment must be the final determinants.

Chlordiazepoxide and diazepam are the only minor tranquilizers usually administered intramuscularly. There is some question as to how completely these drugs are absorbed into the bloodstream via this route, which is generally used only in cases of acute agitation, when they cannot be administered orally. The intravenous route produces relatively immediate peak blood levels; but it must be used with extreme caution, as cardiorespiratory centers in the brain may become depressed.

Although not conclusively demonstrated with lorazepam, central nervous system depression agents and minor tranquilizers tend to augment each other's sedation effects (Gebhart et al., 1969; Madan et al., 1962; Norio et al., 1971; Milner, 1968; Milner, 1970). However, there is some debate on this matter pertinent to ethanol (Reggiani et al., 1968; Hoffer, 1962; Miller, 1963). Therefore, in general, none of these compounds, including lorazepam, should be administered in the presence of pharmacological agents with central nervous system depressant properties. Interactions with other agents are less conclusive, but chlordiazepoxide has been shown to enhance the lethal effects of cholinesterase inhibitors and amphetamines (Gardocki et al., 1966; Weiss & Orzel, 1967). Benzodiazepines have been demonstrated to double levels of diphenylhydantoin (Dilantin®)

and bishydroxycoumarin, the latter producing impaired blood clotting (Vajda et al., 1971; Taylor, 1967). Certainly, more confirmatory investigation is required with respect to interactions between benzodiazepines and other compounds.

PURPORTED LOCI AND MECHANISM OF ACTION

The minor tranquilizers have been used most effectively for nonpsychotic anxiety. The theories of biochemical bases of anxiety are numerous and beyond the scope of this chapter, but one of the more common neurophysiological hypotheses does merit brief consideration: that is, in anxiety states the cerebral cortex receives an excessive number of incoming stimuli via the limbic system, notably the hippocampus (Warburton, 1972; Pribram, 1969). It has been suggested that the benzodiazepines exert the major part of their anxiolytic (anxiety-reducing) action at subcortical levels of the brain. Specifically, they may act by stimulating the cerebral neuronal production of gamma-aminobutyric acid (GABA), an inhibitory neurotransmitter. This inhibitory activity is thought to occur at the level of the limbic system, creating a quiescence of limbic system structures in response to the excessive incoming stimuli (Iwahara et al., 1972; Olds & Olds, 1969; Schallek & Thomas, 1971; Steiner & Hummel, 1968). It is also thought that these agents work directly at the level of the cortex, depressing the effects of purported anxiety-producing stimuli on the cortical neurons.

PRINCIPLES OF USE

Selection of a Component Agent

No evidence suggests that any of the agents mentioned in Table 4–1 is any more or less effective than any other; thus, other factors will influence the selection of one minor tranquilizer over another. For example:
Presence of desired effects.

   1.   The patient has a history of good therapeutic response.
   2.   The drug has a shorter half-life, which is useful in treating a patient with a specific physiological problem.

Absence of undesired effects.   The patient has a history of hypersensitivity.

Contraindications

Absolute.

1. Previous hypersensitivity (allergic reaction) is the *commonly* accepted absolute contraindication.
2. Glaucoma has been mentioned as a contraindication in some cases. Consensus among some ophthalmologists indicates acceptable use of minor tranquilizers if a patient's glaucoma has been evaluated and treated. Glaucoma thus is classified as an absolute contraindication, but may be considered a relative contraindication, and minor tranquilizers may be administered after consultation with and clearance by an ophthalmologist. Physician preference must be the final determinant.
3. Declining central nervous system level of consciousness from intracerebral causes such as tumor or trauma is an absolute contraindication.
4. Declining central nervous system level of consciousness from extracerebral causes (e.g., toxins such as alcohol) is an absolute contraindication. Most persons undergoing alcohol detoxification receive minor tranquilizers to facilitate withdrawal. It is known, however, that ethyl alcohol and the minor tranquilizers can augment the effect on sedation when used together, so the clinician must determine if the two classes of agents should be used concomitantly. At the very least, patients should be cautioned against alcohol intake while on minor tranquilizers. Certainly, they also should be advised against performing any activity requiring alertness and concentration, such as driving a car or operating heavy machinery, while taking minor tranquilizers.

Relative. The factors of physiologic status must be measured against those of side effects (Table 4–2) to determine whether the disadvantages to use of minor tranquilizers outweigh the advantages, and to delineate the physiologic monitoring or evaluation required during the period of prescription.

Indications

Functional psychiatric indications for use of minor tranquilizers are anxiety or anxious depression of mild to moderate severity, unaccompanied by incipient or manifest schizophrenia, incipient or manifest delusions, or hallucinations (Zapletalek et al., 1966; Lehmann & Ban, 1964; Greenblatt & Shader, 1974). The use of minor tranquilizers in organic states such as alcohol withdrawal and convulsive disorders and as muscle relaxants is well known (Bookman and Randall, 1976).

Table 4–2
Side Effects of Minor Tranquilizers

Side Effect	Purported Mechanism of Production
Drowsiness, sedation (Greenblatt & Shader, 1974)	Exact mechanism unknown; presumably effect on reticular activating system or direct depression of corticol neurons; seems to be a dose-related effect
Ataxia (Greenblatt & Shader, 1974)	Exact mechanism unknown; may be secondary to drowsiness and sedation; also apparently a dose-related effect
Paradoxical agitation reaction (Murray, 1962; Ayd, 1962; DiMascio et al., 1970)	Exact mechanism unknown; theories include: 1. Minor-tranquilizer-induced cortical release of previously submerged psychopathology 2. Production of an organic brain syndrome with associated lability of affect and/or a cortical release pattern similar to that described above
Depression-like syndrome (Ryan et al., 1968)	Exact mechanism unknown, but may be depression of cortical neuronal metabolism
Organic brain syndrome (Hall & Joffe, 1972)	Exact mechanism unknown; presumably minor tranquilizer interference with cortical neuronal metabolism

Dosage Regimens

As with the psychotropic classes discussed elsewhere, stature and age will affect dosage. Specifically, those who are slight of stature, younger than 18, or older than approximately 55 should receive one-fourth to one-third the usual dosage.

Equivalence has not been determined for intramuscular and oral administration. Rather than elaborating specific interagent equivalencies, the usual dosage ranges exclusive of age and stature limitations for each of the benzodiazepine minor tranquilizers mentioned in this chapter are listed in Table 4–1.

The regimens are essentially the same for mild anxiety or anxious depression. Conceptually, the regimen should be tailor-made for each patient, depending on his or her individual psychiatric and physiological considerations. For the healthy, average-sized individual in the 18–55-year range, the starting dosages are listed in Table 4–1. Using diazepam as a model, once the starting dose is determined, incremental increases may be approximately 5 mg. every day or every other day, depending on the patient's tolerance to the lowest dose required to produce remission (as long as this dose does not exceed the upper limit of the dosage range). The patient is kept on this dosage for approximately one month, and then

gradually brought down in approximately 5-mg. decrements to the maintenance level (usually one-third to one-fourth of the peak dosage required to
produce remission). Minor tranquilizers should not be withdrawn abruptly
unless this is absolutely necessary. Withdrawal reactions (e.g., anxiety,
nausea, vomiting, diarrhea, insomnia, convulsions) have been reported
(Hollister et al., 1961). The maintenance level continues for approximately
two to six months, barring any unforseen complications.

In administering the minor tranquilizers, the question of once-a-day
versus divided doses must be considered. Because of the relatively long
half-lives and tissue accumulation, diazepam and chlordiazepoxide may
after several days be considered for administration in a once-daily regimen;
or, at the very least, with the bulk of the dosage administered in the
evening before sleep. Lorazepam and oxazepam have shorter half-lives
with little to no tissue accumulation and, therefore, probably should be
administered in divided daily dosages.

If anxiety or anxious depressions occur with incipient or manifest
schizophrenia, incipient or manifest delusions, or hallucinations, the initial
psychopharmacological class of choice is, as noted, major tranquilizers. If
after remission the anxiety or anxious depression remains and is of mild to
moderate severity, a minor tranquilizer may be added. However, the
addition of minor tranquilizers is usually unnecessary. There are no conclusively known drug-drug interaction problems (concentration or otherwise)
requiring dosage changes in combined minor and major tranquilizer regimens, in contrast to the combination of major tranquilizers and tricyclic
antidepressants (see Chapter 5).

SIDE EFFECTS

Table 4–2 lists the more commonly occurring or reported side effects and
their purported mechanism of production (when known or theorized). The
rationale for considering these side effects remains the same as in preceed-
ing chapters. The pre-prescription work-up for minor tranquilizers is
identical to that described for tricyclic antidepressants (see Chapter 5).

REFERENCES

Ayd, F. J. A Critical Appraisal of Chlordiazepoxide. *Journal. Neuropsychiat.*, 1962,
     3:177.
Bookman, P. H., and Randall, L. O. Therapeutic Users of the Benzodiazepines, in
     L. L. Simpson (ed.), *Drug Treatment of Mental Disorders*. Raven Press,
     New York, 1976, pp. 73–90.

DiMascio, A., Shader, R. I., and Giller, D. R. Behavioral Toxicity. Part III: Perceptual-Cognitive Functions; and Part IV: Emotional (Mood) States, in Shader, R. I., and DiMascio, A., *Psychotropic Drug Side Effects: Clinical and Theoretical Perspectives*. Williams and Wilkins, Baltimore, 1970.

Gardocki, J. F., Schuler, M. E., and Goldstein, L. Reconsideration of the Central Nervous System Pharmacology of Amphetamine. II. Influence of Pharmacologic Agents on Cumulative and Total Lethality in Grouped and Isolated Mice. *Toxicol. Appl. Pharmacol.*, 1966, 9:536.

Gebhart, G. F., Plaa, G. L., and Mitchell, C. L. The Effects of Ethanol Alone and in Combination with Phenobarbital, Chlorpromazine, or Chlordiazepoxide. *Toxicol. Appl. Pharmacol.*, 1969, 15:405.

Greenblatt, D. J., and Shader, R. I. *Benzodiazepines in Clinical Practice*. Raven Press, New York, 1974.

Hall, R. C. W., and Joffe, J. R. Aberrant Response to Diazepam: A New Syndrome. *Am. J. Psychiatry*, 1972, 126:738.

Hoffer, A. Lack of Potentiation by Chlordiazepoxide (Librium) of Depression or Excitation Due to Alcohol. *Canad. Med. Assoc. J.*, 1962, 87:920.

Hollister, L. E., Motzenbecker, F. P., and Degan, R. O. Withdrawal Reactions from Chlordiazepoxide (Librium). *Psychopharmacologia*, 1961, 2:63.

Iwahara, S., Oishi, H., Yamazaki, S., and Sakai, K. Effects of Chlordiazepoxide upon Spontaneous Alteration and the Hippocampal Electrical Activity in White Rats. *Psychopharmacologia*, 1972, 24:496.

Lehmann, H. E., and Ban, T. A. Notes from the Log-Book of a Psychopharmacological Research Unit I. *Canad. Psychiat. J.*, 1964, 9:28.

Madan, B. R., Sharma, J. D., and Vyas, D. S. Some Neuropharmacological Actions of Librium. *Ann. Biochem. Exp. Med.*, 1962, 12:221.

Miller, A. I., D'Agostino, A., and Minski, R. Effects of Combined Chlordiazepoxide and Alcohol in Man. *Quart. J. Stud. Alcohol*, 1963, 24:9.

Milner, G. Interaction between Barbiturates, Alcohol, and Some Psychotropic Drugs. *Med. J. Aust.*, 1970, 1:1204.

———. The Effect of Antidepressants and "Tranquilizers" on the Response of Mice to Ethanol. *Brit. J. Pharmacol.*, 1968, 34:370.

Murray, N. Covert Effects of Chlordiazepoxide Therapy. *J. Neuropsychiat.*, 1962, 3:168.

Norio, M., Isoaho, R., and Idanpaan-Heikkila, J. Interaction of Benzodiazepines and Ethanol on Sleeping Time in Rats. *Scand. J. Clin. Lab. Invest.*, 1971, 27 (*supp. 116*):76.

Olds, M. E., and Olds, J. Effects of Anxiety-Relieving Drugs on Unit Discharges in Hippocampus, Reticular Midbrain, and Pre-Optic Area in the Freely Moving Rat. *Int. J. Neuropharmacol.*, 1969, 8:87.

Pribram, K. H. The Neurobehavioral Analysis of the Limbic Forebrain Mechanisms: Revision and Progress Report, in *Lehman Advances in the Study of Behavior*, Vol. 2. Academic Press, New York, 1969.

Reggiani, G., Hurlimann, A., and Theiss, E. Some Aspects of the Experimental and Clinical Toxicology of Chlordiazepoxide, in S. B. D. Baker, J. R. Bossier, and W. Koll (eds.), *Proceedings of the European Society for the Study of*

Drug Toxicity. Vol. 9. Toxicity and Side Effects of Psychotropic Drugs. Excerpta Medica Foundation, Amsterdam, 1968, pp. 79–97.

Ryan, H. F., Merrill, F. B., Scott, G. E., Krebs, R. and Thompson, B. L. Increase in Suicidal Thoughts and Tendencies. Association with Diazepam Therapy. *JAMA*, 1968, *203*:1137.

Schallek, W., and Thomas, J. Effects of Benzodiazepines on Spontaneous Electrical Activity of Subcortical Areas in Brain of Cat. *Arch. Int. Pharmacody.*, 1971, *192*:321.

Steiner, F. A., and Hummel, P. Effects of Nitrazepam and Phenobarbital on Hippocampal and Lateral Geniculate Neurons in the Cat. *Int. J. Neuropharmacol.*, 1968, 7:61.

Taylor, P. J. Hemorrhage while on Anticoagulant Therapy Precipitated by Drug Interaction. *Arizona Med.*, 1967, *24*:697.

Vajda, F. J. E., Prineas, R. H., and Lovell, R. R. H. Interaction between Phenytoin and the Benzodiazepines. *Brit. Med. J.*, 1971, *1*:346.

Warburton, D. M. The Cholinergic Control of Internal Inhibition, in R. A. Boakes and M. S. Halliday (eds.), *Inhibition and Learning*. Academic Press, London, 1972, p. 431.

Weiss, L. R., and Orzel, R. A. Enhancement of Toxicity by Central Depressant Drugs in Rats. *Toxicol. Appl. Pharmacol.*, 1967, *10*:334.

Zapletalek, M., Stonad, M., Komenda, S., Vackova, M., Barborakova, E., Stepanova, M., Hrbek, J., Beran, I., and Siroka, A. Alimenazine, Chlordiazepoxide, Meprobamate, and Placebo in Anxious Depression Therapy. *Activ. Nerv. Sup.*, 1966, 8:437.

CHAPTER 5

Antidepressants

Agents with the potential for reversing certain depressions can be divided into two major categories. The first includes the sympathomimetic group, (amphetamines and methylphenidate [Ritalin®]). The second includes the true antidepressants, the monoamine oxidase inhibitors (MAO inhibitors) and the tricyclic antidepressants. Table 5–1 lists some representative MAO inhibitors and the more commonly prescribed tricyclic antidepressants.

This chapter focuses on tricyclic antidepressants for several major reasons. First, the sympathomimetic amines and methylphenidate produce only transient antidepressant effects secondary to their rapid breakdown to inactive products; they have the potential to worsen or actually cause certain clinical psychiatric conditions; and they have the potential to produce rather severe side effects, including anxiety, depression on withdrawal, an acute paranoid psychosis closely resembling paranoid schizophrenia, and another psychosis similar to Paranoia Vera (Jacobson, 1958; Landman et al., 1958; Robin & Wisenberg, 1958; General Practitioner Research Group, 1964; Hare et al., 1962; Overall et al., 1962).

The MAO inhibitors, because of potential toxicity, require rather extraordinary precautions (Klein & Davis, 1969). Furthermore, many researchers and clinicians argue that the indicated clinical use of the MAO inhibitors is still a matter of speculation.

PERTINENT PHARMACOKINETICS

The pharmacokinetics of tricyclic antidepressants are, in general, similar to those of major tranquilizers in that these antidepressants possess characteristics that favor their absorption into tissues, high lipid solubility, high protein binding, low ionization, and acidic pH.

55

Table 5-1
Antidepressants: Some Commonly Prescribed
MAO Inhibitors and Tricyclic Agents

MAO Inhibitors	Tricyclics
Hydrazines	imipramine (Tofranil®, Presamine®)
isocarboxazid (Marplan®)	desipramine (Pertofrane®, Norpramin®)
phenelzine (Nardil®)	amitriptyline (Elavil®, Endep®)
	nortriptyline (Aventyl®)
Nonhydrazines	protriptyline (Vivactyl®)
tranylcypromine (Parnate®)	doxepin (Sinequan®, Adapin®)

However, probably because of the time required to establish effective tissue or plasma concentrations, therapeutic effect generally cannot be observed for approximately 10 days to three weeks after onset of treatment (Hollister, 1973; Klein and Davis, 1969). Moreover, certain pharmacologic agents, when administered concomitantly, can affect the concentration and/or performance of tricyclics. Major tranquilizers, methylphenidate (Ritlan®), aspirin, and chloramphenicol are believed to increase the plasma concentration of tricyclic antidepressants. Major tranquilizers have been shown to cause a twofold to threefold elevation of tricyclics when administered concurrently (Hollister, 1973; Gram & Overo, 1972). This is an essential fact to remember because major tranquilizers are probably the most common accompanying psychotropic agent to tricyclics. When both are therapeutically indicated, the antidepressant agents must be prescribed in approximately one-third to one-half of the usual dosage. Interestingly enough, instead of the usual 10 days to three weeks required for detection of therapeutic effect with tricyclics alone, generally only three to 10 days are required for such effect when tricyclics are administered with major tranquilizers. The clinician also must be aware of the anticholinergic side effects possibly enhanced by this combination and be especially mindful of the need for a careful assessment of contraindications and close intraprescription monitoring.

Methylphenidate (Ritalin®) also increases the plasma concentration of tricyclics, but the exact amount is not known conclusively (Zeidenberg et al., 1971). The clinician needs to be watchful for potential effects of this combination as well as for effects of an aspirin-tricyclic combination.

Although they may not actually increase the level of catecholamines, thyroid hormones (especially triiodothyronine) may affect the performance of tricyclics, notably imipramine, in females. This hormone is believed to exert its effect by sensitizing the brain receptor sites to endogenous catecholamines. The effectiveness of this combination remains a matter of speculation (Wilson et al., 1970; Feighner et al., 1972).

Oral contraceptives and barbiturates reportedly lower the effective concentrations of tricyclics, notably nortriptyline and desmethylimipramine (Rizzo et al., 1972). It is not clear to what degree concentrations are decreased, but clinicians should be aware of the possible effect of these agents in an inadequate therapeutic response to tricyclics.

PURPORTED MECHANISM OF ACTION

One well-accepted theory offers a biochemical basis for depression: a deficiency of norepinephrine at synapses in the brain (Schildkraut et al., 1967). Speculation as to the correlation between lowered norepinephrine and depression in humans is drawn largely from animal studies. These studies reveal that catecholaminergic neuronal systems, specifically norepinephrine, may play a role in mediating conscious arousal, activation of motility, reward, and reinforcement. All of these elements may be affected in certain depressions. Pharmacological agents that lower the brain concentration of norepinephrine (e.g., the rauwolfia alkaloids) have the potential for producing a depression (Anchor et al., 1955; Ayd, 1958). On the other hand, pharmacological treatment that restores this molecule to an appropriate level for the individual is effective in such depressions.

Let us now examine how each group of antidepressants' agents is believed to elevate the level of norepinephrine. In the brain, the sympathomimetic agents (amphetamines and methylphenidate) produce a secretion of norepinephrine into the synapse and prevent its reuptake into the presynaptic neuron, with consequent elevation of this substance at the synapse. In addition, the amphetamines enhance the sensitivity of the postsynaptic neuron to norepinephrine, thereby increasing the effectiveness of norepinephrine at the postsynaptic neuron (Besson et al., 1971). The MAO-inhibitor antidepressants prevent the intraneuronal catabolism of norepinephrine by monoamine oxidase (MAO), thereby increasing the quantity of the amine available for expulsion into the central synapse (Zeller & Barsky, 1952). Tricyclic antidepressants inhibit the reuptake of norepinephrine into the presynaptic neuron. Because this reuptake is the major route of inactivation of central norepinephrine, interference with this active process increases the bioavailability of the neurotransmitter at the synapse (Figure 5–1) (Alpers & Himwich, 1969; Carlsson et al., 1969).

At this juncture, a point of potential clinical import is worthy of mention. The sympathomimetic agents and true antidepressants are believed to affect the balance of the other centrally secreted biogenic amines, dopamine and 5-hydroxytryptamine (serotonin), in the same manner as norepinephrine. All three amines have been implicated in the production of certain psychoses: dopamine in schizophrenia; norepinephrine and

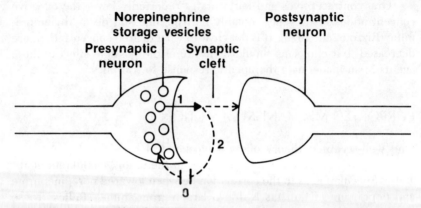

1) Step 1: An electrical impulse traverses the pre-synaptic neuron and causes secretion of norepinephrine from the storage vesicle into the synaptic cleft and activates the post-synaptic neuron.
2) Step 2: After the post-synaptic neuron is activated, norepinephrine is inactivated mainly by its reuptake into the pre-synaptic neuron and subsequent re-storage or catabolism via monamine oxidase.
3) Step 3: The tricyclic antidepressants are believed to exert their predominant therapeutic action by inhibiting step 2, thereby causing an increase in the bioavailability of the amine at the synaptic cleft.

Figure 5–1.   PURPORTED MECHANISM OF THERAPEUTIC ACTION OF TRICY-
CLIC ANTIDEPRESSANTS

dopamine in amphetamine-induced paranoid states; serotonin and dimethylated tryptaminic derivative compounds in psychoses induced by LSD and other hallucinogenic compounds (mescaline and psylocybin) (Snyder et al., 1974). Therefore amphetamines, methylphenidate, MAO inhibitors, and tricyclic antidepressants may not always be used therapeutically. They have the potential, and in some reported cases the demonstrated ability, to make latent and incipient psychoses manifest, to worsen certain existing manifest psychotic states (delusions, hallucinations, and acute schizophrenia) (Pollack et al., 1965; Klein & Davis, 1969; DiMascio & Shader, 1970), and/or to cause mania in predisposed individuals (Bunney et al., 1970; Coppen et al., 1976). In an effort to prevent this unfortunate occurrence, adequate psychiatric assessment (see Chapter 7) must be done before prescribing an antidepressant compound to detect the existence of one of these states in any patient manifesting a depression. With the obvious exception of mania, if one of these syndromes is present as an accompaniment to the depression, major tranquilizers ideally should be prescribed first, with remission produced before the administration of antidepressants.

PRINCIPLES OF USE FOR ANTIDEPRESSANTS

Selection of a Component Drug

To my knowledge, there is no significant difference in therapeutic efficacy among the tricyclic antidepressants listed in Table 5–1. As with the major tranquilizers, however, certain factors, among others, will guide the clinician in selecting one component drug over the other.
Presence of desired effects.

1.　The physician may select a soporific agent useful for a tricyclic antidepressant responsive state that has, as a part of it, a sleep disturbance. (Soporific intensity comparisons are presented in Table 5–2 (Hollister, 1973).

Table 5–2
Relative Comparisons of Tricyclic Antidepressants with Respect to Their Soporific and Anticholinergic Potential (Numerical Values in Increasing Order of Potential)

Tricyclic Agent	Approximate Soporific Potential	Approximate Anticholinergic Potential
protriptyline	1	1
nortriptyline	2	2
desipramine	3	3
imipramine	4	4
amitriptyline	5	5
doxepin	6	6

2.　The patient has a history of good therapeutic response to a drug. If an individual previously responded well to one tricyclic agent, the chance of a similar response to the same or another member of the same class improves (Klein & Davis, 1969; Pare et al., 1962).
Absence of undesired effects.

1.　The patient has a history of a hypersensitivity reaction (allergic).

2.　There is an abnormal physiological state or states that might be worsened by certain pharmacological effect or effects in a particular agent, as in an anticholinergic reaction. Table 5–2 presents comparisons of anticholinergic potential (Klein & Davis, 1969).

Contraindications

Absolute.
1. The patient has a history of a hypersensitivity reaction (allergic).
2. The patient's level of central nervous system consciousness is declining, either from intracerebral causes (e.g., elevation of intracranial pressure) or from extracerebral causes (e.g., barbiturates, alcohol, or other cerebral depressants).

Relative. As with major tranquilizers, the past and current physiological status of the individual must be measured against the potential side effects of the tricyclic antidepressants. For example, assume a 78-year-old man has a history of benign prostatic hypertrophy and urinary hesitancy. Certainly, the physician would wish to avoid the more anticholinergic tricyclics in an effort to preclude worsening the urinary tract problem. Clearance by a cardiologist or internist for prescription of obese agents, as well as monitoring plans, should be obtained in the case of a patient with a history or presence of heart disease.

Indications

The major indication for the use of tricyclic antidepressants is a retarded depression *without* evidence of accompanying incipient or manifest schizophrenia, incipient or manifest delusions, or hallucinations (Kuhn, 1958; Lehmann et al., 1968; Overall et al., 1966). Deviations from this indication might possibly result not only in a lower rate of effectiveness but also in a worsening of the patient's clinical condition. If an organic origin is implicated, appropriate evaluation should establish or negate its presence. If it exists, the treatment of choice, of course, would be reversal of this condition. If it does not exist or cannot be found, tricyclics can be used, but, again, only if there are no absolute or significant contraindications. Physician assessment and judgment are fundamental to these decisions.

Dosage Regimens

As with major tranquilizers, when considering dosage regimens during the acute illness, one must include such components as starting dosage, incremental increases, plateau dosage required to produce remission, decremental decreases to the maintenance level, and the dosage level itself required to maintain remission.

Age. (See discussion for major tranquilizers, Chapter 3.)
Stature. (See discussion for major tranquilizers, Chapter 3.)

Equivalence.   There is little concern over equivalence of antidepressants for the following reasons.

    1.   Tricyclic antidepressants are virtually never administered via the intramuscular route, so there has been no real need to establish equivalence between oral and parenteral routes.

    2.   Only two of the tricyclic antidepressant compounds mentioned in Table 5–1 have been demonstrated to be more potent than the others at the same dosages:

        a.   Protriptyline (Vivactyl®) is approximately five times more potent and, therefore, its dosage range is generally 15–60 mg. per day.

        b.   Nortriptyline (Aventyl®) is approximately two times more potent and, therefore, has a dosage range of around 40–150 mg. per day (Hollister, 1973).

Disease state.   The regimens proposed below are not adjusted for stature, age, or equivalence (in the two cases just noted). Nor are they adjusted for use (when an accompanying pharmacological compound might affect plasma concentration or therapeutic effect).

    1.   At least two types of regimens exist. Begin at 75 mg. of the agent per day either in one or in divided dosages.

        a.   Increase dosage by 75 mg. per week until the desired therapeutic response occurs.

        b.   Increase dosage by 25 mg. every or every other day until the desired therapeutic response occurs.

In either case *DO NOT* exceed 300 mg. per day, first, because therapeutic gains have not been favorable in higher dosages, and second, because the risk of toxicity above 300 mg. per day is considerably higher (Klein & Davis, 1969).

    If 300 mg. does not produce a therapeutic remission of the acute phase within approximately one week, either the medication was not indicated or another treatment form, such as electroconvulsive therapy, should be considered in the absence of contraindications.

    2.   After reaching a therapeutic remission, continue the patient on this dosage for approximately one month, barring unforseen complications.

    3.   Establish a maintenance dosage.

        a.   After one month at remission dosage, begin reducing dosage by approximately 25 mg. a week to the lowest maintenance dosage required to maintain remission.

        b.   *Never abruptly withdraw tricyclics* unless under extreme circumstances, as abrupt withdrawal can result in the same syndrome noted for major tranquilizers.

        c.   Maintenance dosage usually amounts to one-fourth to one-third of the dosage required to produce remission. Maintain patient at this level for approximately six months. It is important to note that these agents, unlike major tranquilizers, have not been conclusively demonstrated to prevent recurrent depressions. This issue must be handled on an individual basis; if at discontinuation of the dosage at the end of a six-month period the patient enters another tricyclic-antidepressant-responsive depression, the practitioner obviously will have to consider a longer maintenance time, once the new episode is brought into remission.

4. Should the patient manifest a retarded depression, accompanied by incipient or manifest schizophrenia, incipient or manifest delusions, or hallucinations, the *initial* drug treatment should be aimed at the accompanying syndrome(s) and not the retarded depression.

   a.   Initially, treat with major tranquilizers until remission of the accompanying syndrome(s), and continue the patient on the appropriate major tranquilizer regimen as discussed in Chapter 3.

   b.   At the time the major tranquilizer-responsive accompanying syndrome is brought into remission, if the retarded depression has persisted, a tricyclic antidepressant can be added at *one-third* the usual dosage.

   c.   Gradually increase the tricyclic antidepressant to the lowest dosage required to produce remission. It is important to remember that while a patient is on a major tranquilizer, the highest dosage of tricyclic antidepressants permissible is approximately 100 mg. (one-third of 300 mg.). If a dosage at 100 mg. fails to produce remission, consider the alternative treatment modalities noted under the standard tricyclic regimens for pure retarded depressions.

   d.   Continue the patient on the remission-producing dosage for approximately one month.

   e.   Gradually decrease the tricyclic to the lowest dosage required to maintain remission and continue the maintenance dosage for approximately six months.

Psychiatric assessment. Psychiatric assessment should precede initiation of tricyclic pharmacotherapy as well as every consideration of change in its therapeutic regimen.

SIDE EFFECTS

Table 5–3 lists the more commonly occurring or reported side effects of tricyclic antidepressants, some of their purported mechanisms of production, and more commonly implicated agents. This list is not intended to discourage prescription of these agents; they can be used effectively for the indicated syndrome. However, they are potentially toxic agents and can disrupt physiological homeostasis. This caveat should, however,

1.   remind the reader that adequate psychiatric assessment should always determine whether the drug is indicated, and that monitoring the agent should continue not only until remission, but also during mainte- nance treatment, and
2.   remind the reader of the necessity for physiological assessment to determine the absolute and relative contraindications to the use of these agents, and the required monitoring during psychopharmacologic treat- ment.

The preantidepressant prescription work-up is the same as for major tranquilizers, except that the T_3 and T_4 are not usually included in this determination. Naturally, if a thyroid abnormality is an etiological consid- eration for the depression, thyroid function tests would be in order. These laboratory tests ideally should be repeated at intervals of approximately six months to one year to monitor intraprescription physiology. Should any interim physiological problem arise before the scheduled repeat of the laboratory battery that might affect further prescription of the tricyclic antidepressant, the appropriate tests should be ordered.

Table 5–3 follows on pages 64 through 67.

Table 5–3
Side Effects of Tricyclic Antidepressants

Side Effects	Purported Mechanism of Production	Commonly Implicated Agents or Groups
I. Vital Signs		
A. *Blood pressure.* Orthostatic hypotension in most cases; severe cases have hypotension in supine position (Muller et al., 1961)	Exact mechanism unknown	More anticholinergic agents, although all have potential
B. *Pulse rate.* Tachycardia	Increased rate probably secondary to hypotension; also, tricyclics can have stimulatory effect on chronotropic mechanisms of heart, possibly due to effect of tricyclic-induced elevated catecholamines	More anticholinergic agents presumably responsible for compensatory tachycardia; however, all have the potential; stimulatory effect not known to be peculiar to one or other of the agents
C. *Temperature* (see X)		
D. *Weight.* increase (Kessler, 1978)	Exact mechanism unknown	Unknown
II. Central Nervous System		
A. *Sedation.* Usually self-limited, ending approximately two to three weeks after final increase of medication	Unknown	More anticholinergic agents, although all have the potential
B. *Organic brain syndrome* (Davies et al., 1971)	Unknown; however, presumably results from interference with cerebro-cortical neuronal metabolism	None specific
C. *Worsening of existing delusions, hallucinations, incipient or manifest schizophrenia, or making incipient delusions manifest* (Angst et al., 1969; Greenblatt & Shader, 1973)	Possibly secondary to central anticholinergic effect, as with major tranquilizers, the depression of acetylcholine producing a rise in dopamine in the brain; also tricyclic-induced elevation of biogenic amines	More anticholinergic agents in the first case; however, all have the potential in both the first and second cases

64

D. *Lowering of seizure threshold*	Exact mechanism unknown	None specific
E. *Extrapyramidal disorders.* Can make latent tardive dyskinesia manifest (Tarsy & Baldessarini, 1976)	By elevating central dopamine in relation to acetylcholine, presumably secondary to lowering acetylcholine at the level of the basal ganglia, the theorized mechanism discussed in Chapter 3	More anticholinergic agents, although all have the potential
F. *Fine tremor of upper extremities* (Klerman & Cole, 1965)	Exact mechanism unknown	All have the potential
G. *Sweating of head and neck* (Shader & Harmatz, 1970)	Effect on superior cervical ganglion, mechanism unknown	Imipramine and doxepin, but probably all have the potential
III. Eyes		
A. *Blurring of vision* (Appleton, 1970; Kessler, 1978)	Anticholinergic-induced mydriasis	More anticholinergic agents, although all have the potential
B. *Decreased accommodation*	Same	Same
C. *Elevation of intraocular pressure*	Anticholinergic-induced mydriasis, causing impingement on canal of Schlemm, producing problems with egress of intraocular fluid from anterior chamber of eye	More anticholinergic agents, although all have the potential
IV. Nose		
Nasal dryness, stuffiness	Anticholinergic-induced drying of secretions in mucosa	Same
V. Mouth		
Dryness with occasional thirst; occasional reports of moniliasis (Angst & Theobald, 1970; Everett, 1975)	Same as with major tranquilizers	Same

Table 5-3 (continued)
Side Effects of Tricyclic Antidepressants

Side Effects	Purported Mechanism of Production	Commonly Implicated Agents or Groups
VI. Heart		
T-Wave flattening and inversion; lengthening of P-R interval; tachycardia; lengthening of QRS complex; lengthening of Q-T interval; second degree or complete A-V block; ventricular arrhythmias (ventricular premature depolarization, ventricular tachycardia, ventricular fibrillation); atrial arrhythmias (atrial tachycardia, atrial flutter, atrial fibrillation) (Kristiansen, 1961; Rasmussen & Kristjansen, 1963; Vohra et al., 1975; Josephson et al., 1974; Barnes et al., 1968; Freeman et al., 1969; Noble & Matthew, 1969; Rasmussen, 1965; Williams & Sherter, 1971; Sigg et al., 1963; Langslet et al., 1971; Muller & Burckhardt, 1974)	Exact mechanism unknown; however, retarded conduction disturbances may be due to either depressed myocardial contractibility, direct myocardial depression, quinidine-like effect or cholinergic blockade; accelerated or irregular conduction may be secondary to sympathomimetic activity	Most have been implicated, but all have the potential; specifics are still under investigation
VII. Abdomen **(Klein & Davis, 1969)**		
A. *Gastrointestinal tract.* Constipation	Anticholinergic-induced hypoperistalsis	More anticholinergic agents, although all have the potential
B. *Liver.* Various degrees of an acute hepatitic-like syndrome, including malaise, lassitude, nausea, vomiting, abdominal pain, hepatomegaly, jaundice, pruritis, and abnormalities in one or more liver function tests (SGOT, SGPT, total/direct bilirubin, alkaline phosphatase)	Allergic hypersensitivity reaction with accumulation of eosinophils in small bile ducts of liver, producing a cholestatic obstruction and consequent clinical complex	None specific

66

VIII. Genitourinary Tract

A. *Urinary Tract.* Urinary hesitancy or retention (Merrill & Markland, 1970)	Presumably from anticholinergic effect	More anticholinergic agents, although all have the potential
B. *Reproductive Tract.*		
1. *Female.* Amenorrhea and irregular menses (Kessler, 1978)	Exact mechanisms unknown	None specific
2. *Male.* Orgasmic or ejaculatory dysfunction (absent or delayed) (Couper-Smartt & Rodham, 1973)	Exact mechanism unknown	More anticholinergic agents, although all have the potential

IX. Skin

Systemic reaction	Allergic hypersensitivity, exact mechanism unknown	All have the potential

X. Hematopoietic System

Agranulocytosis, manifested by elevated temperature and sore throat; pharyngeal inspection usually reveals erythema and ulcerations, and the c.b.c. shows a decline and/or significant reduction to only a few white cells, specifically neutrophils; may occur at any time in treatment, but usually occurs between sixth and eighth week of therapy; any evidence of sore throat and/or elevated temperature requires immediate c.b.c. with differential and serial c.b.c.s with differential, as indicated, regardless of the duration of tricyclic antidepressant treatment (Bird, 1960)	Exact mechanism unknown	All have the potential

REFERENCES

Anchor, R. W. P., Hanson, N. O., and Gifford, R. W. Hypertension Treated with Rauwolfia Serpentina (Whole Root) and with Reserpine: Controlled Study Disclosing Occasional Severe Depression. *JAMA*, 1955, *159*:841.

Alpers, H. S., and Himwich, H. An in Vitro Study of the Effects of Tricyclic Antidepressant Drugs on the Accumulation of C^{14}-Serotonin by Rabbit Brain. *Biol. Psychiatry*, 1969, *1*:81.

Angst, J., Dittrich, A., and Grof, P. Course of Endogenous Affective Psychoses and Its Modification by Prophylactic Administration of Imipramine and Lithium. *Int. Pharmacopsychiat.*, 1969, *2*:1.

Angst, J., and Theobaid, W. *Tofranil (Imipramine)*. Verlag Stampfli and Cie, Berne, 1970.

Appleton, W. S. Skin and Eye Complications of Psychoactive Drug Therapy, In DiMascio, A., and Shader, R. I. (eds.), *Clinical Handbook of Psychopharmacology*. Jason Aronson, New York, 1970.

Ayd, F. J., Drug-Induced Depression—Fact or Fallacy? *N.Y. State J. Med.*, 1958, *58*:354.

Barnes, R. J., Kong, S. M., and Wu, R. W. Y. Electrocardiographic Changes in Amitriptyline Poisoning. *Brit. Med. J.*, 1968, *3*:222.

Besson, M., Cheramy, A., Feltz, P., and Glowinski, J. Dopamine: Spontaneous and Drug Induced Release from the Caudate Nucleus in the Cat. *Brain Res.*, 1971, *32*:407.

Bird, C. E. Agranulocytosis Due to Imipramine (Tofranil). *Canad. Med. Assn. J.*, 1960, *82*:1021.

Bunney, W. E., Jr., Murphy, D. L., Brodie, H., and Goodwin, F. K. L-Dopa in Depressed Patients. *Lancet*, 1970, *1*:352.

Carlsson, A., Corrodi, H., Fuxe, K., and Holfelt, T. Effect of Antidepressant Drugs on the Depletion of Intraneuronal Brain 5-Hydroxytryptamine Stores Caused by 4-Methyl-α-Ethyl-Meta-Tyramine. *Eur. J. Pharmacol.*, 1969, *5*:357.

Coppen, A., Montgomery, S. A., Gupta, R. K., and Bailey, J. E. A Double-Blind Comparison of Lithium Carbonate and Maprotiline in the Prophylaxis of the Affective Disorders. *Brit. J. Psychiat.*, 1976, *128*:479.

Couper-Smartt, J. D., and Rodham, R. A Technique for Surveying Side-Effects of Tricyclic Drugs with Reference to Reported Sexual Effects. *J. Int. Med. Res.*, 1973, *1*:473.

Davies, R. K., Tucker, G. J., Harrow, M., and Detre, T. P. Confusional Episodes and Antidepressant Medication. *Amer. J. Psychiat.*, 1971, *128*:127.

DiMascio, A., and Shader, R. I. (eds.). *Clinical Handbook of Psychopharmacology: Behavioral Toxicity*. Jason Aronson, New York, 1970.

Everett, H. C. The Use of Bethanecol Chloride with Tricyclic Antidepressants. *Am. J. Psychiat.*, 1975, *132*:1202.

Feighner, J. P., King, L. J., Schukit, M. A., Croughan, J., and Briscoe, W.

Hormonal Potentiation of Imipramine and ECT in Primary Depression. *Am. J. Psychiat.*, 1972, *128*:1230.

Freeman, J. W., Mundy, G. R., Beattie, R. R., and Ryan, C. Cardiac Abnormalities in Poisoning with Tricyclic Antidepressants. *Brit. Med. J.*, 1969, *2*:610.

General Practitioner Research Group. Report Number 51. Dexamphetamine Compared with an Inactive Placebo in Depression. *Practitioner*, 1964, *192*:151.

Gram, L. F., and Overo, K. F. Drug Interaction: Inhibitory Effect of Neuroleptics on Metabolism of Tricyclic Antidepressants in Man. *Br. Med. J.*, 1972, *1*:463.

Greenblatt, D. J., and Shader, R. I. Drug Therapy: Anticholinergics. *N. Engl. J. Med.*, 1973, *288*:1215.

Hare, E. H., Dominian, J., and Sharpe, L. Phenelzine and Dexamphetamine in Depressive Illness: A Comparative Trial. *Brit. Med. J.*, 1962, *1*:9.

Hollister, L. E. *Clinical Use of Psychotherapeutic Drugs*, Charles C Thomas, Springfield, Ill., 1973.

Jacobson, A. The Use of Ritalin in Psychotherapy of Depression of the Aged. *Psychiat. Quart.*, 1958, *32*:474.

Josephson, M. E., Seides, S. F., Batsford, W. P., Weisfogel, G. M., Akhtar, M., Caracta, A. R., Lau, S. H., and Damato, A. N. The Electrophysiological Effects of Intramuscular Quinidine on the Atrioventricular Conducting System in Man. *Am. Heart. J.*, 1974, *87*:55.

Kessler, K. A. Tricyclic Antidepressants: Made of Action and Clinical Use, in Lipton, M. A., DiMascio, A., and Killam, K. F. (eds.), *Psychopharmacology: A Generation of Progress*. Raven Press, New York, 1978.

Klein, D. F., and Davis, J. M. *Diagnosis and Drug Treatment of Psychiatric Disorders*. Williams and Wilkins, Baltimore, 1969.

Klerman, G., and Cole, J. O. Clinical Pharmacology of Imipramine and Related Antidepressant Compounds. *Pharmacol. Rev.*, 1965, *17*:101.

Kristiansen, E. S. Cardiac Complications during Treatment with Imipramine (Tofranil). *Acta. Psychiatr. Neurol. Scand.*, 1961, *36*:427.

Kuhn, R. The Treatment of Depressive States with G22355 (Imipramine Hydrochloride). *Am. J. Psychiat.*, 1958, *115*: 459.

Landman, M. E., Preisig, R., and Perlman, M. Practical Mood Stimulant. *J. Med. Soc.*, New Jersey, 1958, *55*:155.

Langslet, A., Johansen, W. G., Ryg, M., Skomedal, T., and Oye, I. Effects of Dibenzepine and Imipramine on the Isolated Rat Heart. *Eur. J. Pharmacol.*, 1971, *14*:333.

Lehmann, H. E., Cahn, C. H., and DeVerteuil, R. L. The Treatment of Depressive Conditions with Imipramine (G22355). *Can. Psychiat. Assoc. J.*, 1968, *3*:155.

Merrill, D. C., and Markland, C. Vesical Dysfunction Induced by the Major Tranquilizers. *J. Urol.*, 1972, *107*:769.

———. A Laboratory Investigation of the Effect of Phenothiazines on Urinary Bladder Function. *Invest. Urol.*, 1970, 7:532.

Muller, O. E., Goodman, N., and Bellett, S. The Hypotensive Effect of Imipramine Hydrochloride in Patients with Cardiovascular Disease. *Clin. Pharmacol. Ther.*, 1961, 2:300.

Muller, V., and Burckhardt, D. Die Wirkung Tri- und Tetrazyklischer Antidepresiva auf Herz und Kreislauf. *Schweiz Med. Wschr.*, 1974, 104:1911.

Noble, J., and Matthew, H. Acute Poisoning by Tricyclic Antidepressants: Clinical Features and Management of 100 Patients. *Clin. Toxicol.*, 1969, 2:403.

Overall, J. E., Hollister, L. E., Johnson, J., and Pennington, V. Nosology of Depression and Differential Response to Drugs. *JAMA*, 1966, 195:946.

Overall, J. E., Hollister, L. E., Pokorny, A. D., Casey, J. F., and Katz, G. Drug Therapy in Depressions. Controlled Evaluation of Imipramine Isocarboxazid, Dextroamphetamine-Amobarbital, and Placebo. *Clin. Pharmacol. Ther.*, 1962, 3:16.

Pare, C. M. B., Rees, L., and Sainsbury, M. J. Differentiation of Two Genetically Specific Types of Depression by the Response to Antidepressants. *Lancet*, 1962, 2:1340.

Pollack, M., Klein, D. F., Willner, A., Blumberg, A. G., and Fink, M. Imipramine Induced Behavioral Disorganization in Schizophrenic Patients. Physiological and Psychological Correlates. *Recent Advances Biol. Psychiat.*, 1965, 7:53.

Rasmussen, E. B., and Kristjansen, P. ECG Changes during Amitriptyline Treatment. *Am. J. Psychiat.*, 1963, 119:781.

Rasmussen, J. Amitriptyline and Imipramine Poisoning. *Lancet*, 1965, 2:850.

Rizzo, M., Pantarotto, C., Riva, E., Gianelli, A., Morselli, P. L., and Garattini, S. Interactions of Tricyclic Antidepressants with Other Drugs. Paper read at Fifth International Congress of Pharmacology, San Francisco, 1972.

Robin, A. A., and Wisenberg, S. A Controlled Trial of Methylphenidate (Ritalin) in the Treatment of Depressive States. *J. Neurol. Neurosurg. Psychiat.*, 1958, 21:55.

Schildkraut, J. J., Schanberg, S. M., Breese, G. R., and Kopin, I. J. Norepinephrine Metabolism and Drugs Used in the Affective Disorders: A Possible Mechanism of Action. *Am. J. Psychiat.*, 1967, 124:54.

Shader, R. I., and Harmatz, J. S. Gastrointestinal Effects, in Shader, R. I., and DiMascio, A. (eds.), *Psychotropic Drug Side Effects*. Robert E. Krieber, Huntington, N.Y., 1970.

Sigg, E. B., Osborne, M., and Korol, B. Cardiovascular Effects of Imipramine. *J. Pharmacol. Exp. Ther.*, 1963, 141:237.

Snyder, S. H., Banerjee, S. P., Yamamura, H. I., and Greenberg, D. Drugs, Neurotransmitters, and Schizophrenia. *Science*, 1974, 184:1243.

Tarsy, D., and Baldessarini, R. J. The Tardive Dyskinesia Syndrome, in Klawans, H. (ed.), *Clinical Neuropharmacology*. Raven Press, New York, 1976, pp. 29–61.

Vohra, J., Burrows, G. D., and Sloman, G. Assessment of Cardiovascular Side Effects of Therapeutic Doses of Tricyclic Antidepressant Drugs. *Aust. N. Z. J. Med.*, 1975, 5:7.

Williams, R. B., and Sherter, C. Cardiac Complications of Tricyclic Antidepressant Therapy. *Ann. Intern. Med.*, 1971, *74*:395.

Wilson, I. C., Prange, A. J., McClane, T. K., Rabon, A. M., and Lipton, M. A. Thyroid-Hormone Enhancement of Imipramine in Nonretarded Depressions. *New Eng. J. Med.*, 1970, *282*:1063.

Zeidenberg, P., Perel, J. M., Kanzler, M., Wharton, R. N., and Malitz, S. Clinical and Metabolic Studies with Imipramine in Man. *Am. J. Psychiat.*, 1971, *127*:1321.

Zeller, E. A., and Barsky, J. In Vivo Inhibition of Liver and Brain Monoamine Oxidase by 1-isonicotinyl-2-isopropylhydrazine. *Proc. Soc. Exp. Biol. Med.*, 1952, *81*:459.

CHAPTER 6

Lithium

Depression falls at one pathological extreme of the mood and affect spectrum. The opposite extreme, euphoria and elation (Hypomania and mania), is considered in this chapter. The most commonly used agent for hypomania and mania is lithium, administered in the carbonate salt form.

PERTINENT PHARMACOKINETICS

Lithium, the lightest known metal, is administered orally. It is absorbed fairly rapidly through the intestinal mucosa; peak blood levels are attained in approximately one to two hours. Lithium requires from six to 10 days from first administration for sufficient uptake into the brain to initiate a therapeutic response. After the patient has been receiving the agent for a while, the half-life is approximately 18–36 hours, with the longer half-life probably occurring in patients with suboptimal metabolic integrity. Lithium is excreted primarily by the kidneys. Therefore, circulatory competence is required to avoid undue time lag in the body and subsequent complications of toxicity from abnormally high serum and tissue concentrations (Jefferson & Greist, 1977; Caldwell et al., 1971; Hollister, 1973; Bunney, 1968; Klein & Davis, 1969; Gershon, 1974).

Of potential clinical significance is the fact that intracellular sodium ions deter absorption of lithium ions into the cell. Thus, if total body sodium is low, the low intracellular concentration of sodium ions will produce an increased cellular reabsorption of lithium and increase the risk of lithium toxicity. The sodium-lithium ionic exchange normally occurs in the kidney (Thomsen & Schou, 1968).

PURPORTED LOCI AND MECHANISM OF ACTION

There is no clear consensus regarding possible biochemical origins of mania and hypomania, but one of the most popular theories suggests an increase in norepinephrine at the central synapse, a mechanism opposite that of certain depressions. Therefore, unlike antidepressants, lithium is believed to work by reducing norepinephrine to a normal level. Theoretically, lithium causes an increased reuptake of norepinephrine into the presynaptic neuron, thereby decreasing the concentration of the biogenic amine at the synaptic cleft (Hollister, 1973; Gerbino et al., 1978).

PRINCIPLES OF USE

Contraindications

Absolute.
    1.   The patient has had a previous allergic reaction to lithium.
    2.   The patient suffers from cardiovascular or renal disease of sufficient magnitude to dangerously retard lithium excretion from the body.
Relative.   The relative contraindications are essentially the same for lithium carbonate as for major tranquilizers and antidepressants. The patient's past and current physiological statuses are measured against the potential side effects of lithium. The decision to prescribe lithium will include consideration of special clearances from other appropriate specialists and/or monitoring.

Two major types of side effects, idiosyncratic and dose-related, may contraindicate use. Idiosyncratic side effects listed in Table 6–1 should be taken into careful consideration before prescription. Dose-related side effects, which can be monitored relatively well with regular tests of serum lithium concentration and clinical observation, are not likely to occur unless the serum concentrations of the ion approach toxic levels. The patient's physiological capacity to excrete the ion should be considered, with appropriate regimen adjustments and monitoring.

Because there is only one member of this psychotropic drug class, selection of one agent over the other naturally is not a consideration.

Table 6-1
Side Effects of Lithium

Side Effects	Purported Mechanism of Production
Dose Related[a]	
(Vancaflor, 1975; Schou et al., 1970; Shopsin et al., 1970; Branchey et al., 1976; Mayfield & Brown, 1966; Johnson et al., 1970; Reilly et al., 1973; Baldessarini & Stephens, 1970; Demers et al., 1970)	
Lethargy, sluggishness, patient dazed, muscle twitchings, hand tremor (fine or coarse)	Presumably effect of lithium on central nervous system, although exact mechanism unknown
Extrapyramidal signs (predominantly parkinsonism)	Same
EEG abnormalities	Same
Seizures	Same
Increased muscle tone	Same
Nausea, vomiting, abdominal pain	Unknown
Polyuria	Unknown
Excessive thirst	Unknown
Coma	Presumably effect of lithium on central nervous system
Death (usually from intercurrent pulmonary infection)	
Nondose Related (Idiosyncratic)[b]	
(Gershon, 1970; Goldfield & Weinstein, 1971; Kusumi, 1971; Schou, 1968; Shopsin et al., 1971)	
Organic brain syndrome; usually reversible off lithium	Lithium effect on cortical neurons; exact mechanism unknown
Hashimoto's-disease-like syndrome with diffuse thyroid enlargement; usually without disturbance of thyroid function, but there are some reports of hypothyroidism	Unknown
Diabetes-insipidus-like syndrome with polyuria and excessive thirst	Unknown
Leukocytosis (as high as 20,000 cells per cubic milliliter or slightly greater)	Unknown
Teratogenic effects	Unknown
Skin eruptions; begin as acneiform papules that may erupt, coalesce, and/or spread	Unknown
Flattening or inversion of T-wave on EKG	Unknown

[a]Because these side effects are dose-related, they should be corroborated at once by serum lithium determination.
[b]Most of these are believed to be reversible with termination of the drug. However, in the case of an organic brain syndrome, if cortical neuronal metabolism is impaired either long or extensively enough, presumably irreversible damage may be done.

Indications

Acute states. Lithium is indicated for acute mania/hypomania (without
the presence of incipient or manifest schizophrenia,* incipient or manifest
delusions, or hallucinations) (Fann et al., 1969; Schou, 1963; Maggs, 1963;
Fieve et al., 1969; Pokorny & Prien, 1974; Johnson et al., 1971; Prien et al.,
1972b; Johnson et al., 1968; Spring et al., 1970; Davis & Fann, 1971). It is
under investigation for potential use for schizophrenia (schizo-affective,
excited or manic subtype); certain depressions (usually retarded types);
epileptoid, aggressive, or emotionally unstable personality disorders; alcoholism; and premenstrual tension (Annell, 1969; Frommer, 1968; Sheard,
1971; Merry et al., 1976; Rifkin et al., 1972; Sletten & Gershon, 1966;
Fries, 1969; Gershon, 1974; Schou, 1968). Use for any but the major
indications may risk not only lowered or no therapeutic response, but also
toxicity; lithium is not an innocuous agent. However, close attention
should be given to new work regarding the effects of lithium on these other
potentially severe disorders.
Maintenance states. Lithium acts as a prophylaxis against recurrent acute
mania or hypomania (without accompanying incipient or manifest schizophrenia, incipient or manifest delusions, or hallucinations) (Noack &
Trautner, 1951; Gershon & Yuwiler, 1960). It has been suggested for use in
recurrent mania or hypomania alternating with depression, and in recurrent depressions, all of which are more speculative uses (Baastrup et al.,
1970; Prien et al., 1973; Prien et al., 1974).

Dosage Regimens

Age. Appropriate reductions in dosages must be made for patients
younger than about 18 years of age (although it is unlikely for acute mania
or hypomania to occur at this early age) and for patients older than about
55.
Stature. Dosage reductions should be made for patients of small stature,

---

*"Manifest schizophrenia" includes all clinical subtypes of this diagnostic entity. It is especial-
ly difficult for some to differentiate clinically the catatonic-excited subtype of schizophrenia
from acute mania or hypomania. This has significant therapeutic implications, since lithium is
not useful therapeutically in the former state. Confusion in this differentiation rests usually
with increased motor activity, which is present in both. However, the activity is more
purposeful in acute mania and hypomania (as opposed to erratic and rage-like activity in the
catatonic-excited state). Further, unlike the schizophrenic state, acute mania and hypomania
are accompanied by elation and pressure of speech and thought.

but should *not* be increased for larger individuals. For both age and size, reduce the usual starting dosage by two-thirds. It is always possible to increase the dosage, but is sometimes quite difficult to undo physiological harm from dosage excess.

Equivalence. Obviously, equivalence need not be considered, as there is no intramuscular administration, and lithium carbonate is the sole member of its group currently in common use.

Disease States. The following are general guidelines for patients who do not require any dosage adjustments described above.

  1. Average starting dosage is 300 mg. three times daily.

  2. Dosage is increased by 300 mg. every day or every other day until the desired therapeutic response occurs. This is true even with reduced starting doses.

  3. Unlike major-tranquilizer and antidepressant regimens, once the dosage required to produce remission is met, reduction in dosage must begin. (As the patient enters remission, the brain, it is believed, utilizes less lithium, causing an increase in plasma concentration and consequent higher risk of toxicity [Jefferson & Greist, 1977]).

    a. Withdraw patient gradually to the lowest dosage required to maintain remission.

    b. Usually, reduce dosage by 300 mg. every several days.

    c. Lithium carbonate can be discontinued abruptly in an emergency situation.

  4. Usual maintenance dosage level is approximately one-third of the dosage required to produce remission.

  5. Duration of maintenance treatment is under debate. The theoretical camps are divided with respect to first-occurrence episode of the illness. Many agree that after a relatively short period on the maintenance dosage, the patient may be withdrawn gradually, with careful counseling of the patient and family about symptoms and signs of recurrence that require professional help. Consensus tends toward lifetime maintenance treatment after a second occurrence.

  6. If acute mania or hypomania is accompanied by incipient or manifest schizophrenia, the psychopharmacological treatment of choice is major tranquilizers. Lithium has been shown to be less effective in these cases and, in some instances with acute mania or hypomania accompanied by acute schizophrenia (schizophrenia, schizo-affective, excited or manic subtype), has been shown to cause a worsening in clinical status of the patient.

  7. If acute mania or hypomania occurs with incipient or manifest delusions or hallucinations, lithium carbonate should be used for the mania or hypomania, and major tranquilizers should be prescribed for the other

symptoms, in a regimen as described in Chapter 3. Note that there is some
concern that lithium in combination with haloperidol (Haldol®) can produce an irreversible organic brain syndrome, although this still seems to be
a matter of debate (Cohen & Cohen, 1974; Marhold et al., 1974; Ayd,
1975).

DETERMINATION OF SERUM CONCENTRATION

In prescribing lithium, a required determination is the serum lithium
concentration (measured in milliequivalents [mEq.] per liter), because
lithium is the only psychotropic agent that demonstrates a good correlation
between blood level and therapeutic response, as well as dose-related side
effects. This serum concentration is usually measured shortly before the
first lithium carbonate dose of the morning (or approximately eight to 12
hours after the last dose of the preceding day), as this corresponds to its
original method of standardization. Serum lithium concentrations should
ideally be measured:

1   before initiating a new lithium regimen, if the patient previously
has been on the medication (although the serum concentration falls by
one-half each day after discontinuation of the drug),
2.   before an increase in dosage during the acute phase of the illness,
3.   before a dosage decrease, and
4.   at the first symptom or sign of clinical therapeutic worsening or
toxicity.

During the acute-illness phase of treatment (including starting dosage,
incremental stage, and decremental stage to maintenance levels), the
serum lithium determinations should probably be done every day or every
other day. Once a patient is relatively stabilized at the maintenance level,
these measurements generally may be made less frequently, barring any
unforeseen complications. However, they should be done at least every
month.

The serum lithium determination does not substitute for clinical
assessment (by interview), which ideally should be done daily during the
acute stage and certainly before any change in dosage regimen is im-
plemented. It is not uncommon to find an individual approaching the
acute-stage therapeutic range (0.8–1.4 mEq./l.) (Prien et al., 1972a) and
not yet in clinical remission. Nor is it impossible to see a patient not yet at
the appropriate therapeutic level but nevertheless nearing clinical remis-

sion. The therapeutic range for the maintenance of remission is approximately 0.2 to 0.9 mEq./l.; however, clinical opinion differs (Jefferson & Greist, 1977). Close assessment for status of the remission and toxicity remains one of the best guides, insuring, however, that the serum concentration does not exceed 1.4 mEq./l.

The serum lithium concentration is a key factor in predicting the likelihood of dose-related side effects. The incidence of these effects increases at serum lithium concentrations of greater than 1.4 mEq./l.; these effects can, however, occur at lower concentrations. Therefore, serum lithium levels should always be checked if there is any question about the appearance of side effects.

SIDE EFFECTS

Table 6–1 lists the most commonly occurring or reported dose-related and idiosyncratic side effects of lithium as well as some purported mechanisms of their production.

The rationale for their delineation is the same as that noted in Chapters 3 and 5. The prelithium carbonate prescription work-up is also the same as for major tranquilizers.

REFERENCES

Annell, A. L. Manic-Depressive Illness in Children and Effect of Treatment with Lithium Carbonate. *Acta Paedopsychiatr.*, 1969, *36*:292.

Ayd, F. J. Lithium-Haloperidol for Mania: Is It Safe or Hazardous? *Int. Drug Ther. Newsletter.*, 1975, *10*:29.

Baastrup, P. C., Poulsen, J. C., Schou, M., Thomsen, K., and Amidsen, A. Prophylactic Lithium: Double Blind Discontinuation in Manic Depressive and Recurrent Depressive Disorders. *Lancet*, 1970, *2*:326.

Baldessarini, R. J., and Stephens, J. H. Lithium Carbonate for Affective Disorders. I. Clinical Pharmacology and Toxicology. *Arch. Gen. Psychiatr.*, 1970, *22*:72.

Branchey, M. H., Charles, J., and Simpson, G. M. Extrapyramidal Side Effects in Lithium Maintenance Therapy. *Am. J. Psychiatr.*, 1976, *133*:444.

Bunney, W. E., Goodwin, F. K., Davis, J. M., and Fawcett, J. A. A Behavioral-Biochemical Study of Lithium in Therapy. *Am. J. Psychiatr.*, 1968, *125*:91.

Caldwell, H. C., Westlake, W. J., Connor, S. M., and Flanagen, T. A Pharmacokinetic Analysis of Lithium Carbonate Absorption from Several Formulations in Man. *J. Clin. Pharmacol.*, 1971, *11*:349.

Cohen, W. J., and Cohen, N. H. Lithium Carbonate, Haloperidol, and Irreversible Brain Damage, *JAMA*, 1974, *230*:1283.

Davis, J. M., and Fann, W. E. Lithium. *Annual Review of Pharmacology*, 1971, *11*:285.

Demers, R., Ludesh, R., and Pritchard, I. Convulsions during Lithium Therapy. *Lancet*, 1970, *2*:315.

Fann, W. E., Asher, H., and Luton, F. H. Use of Lithium in Mania. *Dis. Nerv. Syst.*, 1969, *30*:605.

Fieve, R. R., Platman, S. R., and Fleiss, J. L. A Clinical Trial of Methysergide and Lithium in Mania. *Psychopharmacologia*, 1969, *15*:425.

Fries, H. Experience with Lithium Barbonate Treatment at a Psychiatric Department in the Period 1964–1967. *Acta. Psychiatr. Scand. Suppl.*, 1969, *207*:41.

Frommer, E. A. Depressive Illness in Childhood, in A. Coppen and A. K. Walk (eds.), *Recent Development in Affective Disorders*. Heady Brothers, 1968, pp. 117–136.

Gerbino, L., Oleshansky, M., and Gershon, S. Clinical Use and Mode of Action of Lithium, in M. A. Lipton, A. DiMascio and K. F. Killam (eds.), *Psychopharmacology: A Generation of Progress*. Raven Press, New York, 1978, pp. 1261–1275.

Gershon, S. Lithium Prophylaxis in Recurrent Affective Disorders. *Compr. Psychiatr.*, 1974, *15*:365.

————, Lithium in Mania. *Clin. Pharmacol. Ther.*, 1970, *11*:168.

Gershon, S., and Yuwiler, A. Lithium Ion: A Specific Psychopharmacological Approach to the Treatment of Mania. *J. Neuropsychiatr.*, 1960, *1*:229.

Goldfield, M., and Weinstein, M. R. Lithium in Pregnancy: A Review with Recommendations. *Am. J. Psychiatr.*, 1971, *127*:888.

Hollister, L. E. *Clinical Use of Psychotherapeutic Drugs*. Charles C Thomas, Springfield, Ill., 1973.

Jefferson, J. W., and Greist, J. H. *Primer of Lithium Therapy*. Williams and Wilkins, Baltimore, 1977.

Johnson, G., Gerson, S., Burdock, E. I., Floyd, A., and Hekemian, L. Comparative Effects of Lithium and Chlorpromazine in the Treatment of Acute Manic States. *Brit. J. Psychiatr.*, 1971, *119*:267.

Johnson G., Gerson, S., and Hekemian, L. J. Controlled Evaluation of Lithium and Chlorpromazine in the Treatment of Manic States: An Interim Report. *Compr. Psychiatr.*, 1968, *9*:563.

Johnson, G., Maccario, M., Gershon, S., and Korein, J. The Effect of Lithium on Electroencephalogram, Behavior and Serum Electrolytes. *J. Nerv. Ment. Dis.*, 1970, *151*:273.

Klein, D. F., and Davis, J. M. *Diagnosis and Drug Treatment of Psychiatric Disorders*. Williams and Wilkins, Baltimore, 1969.

Kusumi, Y. A Cutaneous Side Effect of Lithium: Report of Two Cases. *Dis. Nerv. Syst.*, 1971, *32*:853.

Maggs, R. Treatment of Manic Illness with Lithium Carbonate. *Brit. J. Psychiatr.*, 1963, *109*:56.

Marhold, J., Zimanova, J., Lachman, M., Kral, J., and Vojtechovsky, M. To the

Incompatibility of Haloperidol with Lithium Salts. *Act. Nerv. Super.*, 1974, *16*:199.

Mayfield, D., and Brown, R. G. The Clinical Laboratory and Electroencephalographic Effects of Lithium. *J. Psychiatr. Res.*, 1966, *4*:207.

Merry, J., Reynolds, C. M., Bailey, J., and Coppen, A. Prophylactic Treatment of Alcoholism by Lithium Carbonate. *Lancet*, 1976, *2*:481.

Noack, C. H., and Trautner, E. M. The Lithium Treatment of Maniacal Psychosis. *Med. J. Aust.*, 1951, *2*:219.

Pokorny, A. D., and Prien, R. F. Lithium in Treatment and Prevention of Affective Disorder. A VA-NIMH Collaborative Study. *Dis. Nerv. Syst.*, 1974, *35*:327.

Prien, R. F., Caffey, E. M., Jr., and Klett, C. J. Prophylactic Efficacy of Lithium Carbonate in Manic-Depressive Illness: Report of the Veterans Administration and National Institute of Mental Health Collaborative Study Group. *Arch. Gen. Psychiatr.*, 1973, *28*:337.

Prien, R. F., Caffey, E. M., Jr., and Klett, C. J. Factors Associated with Treatment Success in Lithium Carbonate Prophylaxis: Reports of the Veterans Administration and National Institute of Mental Health Collaborative Study Group. *Arch. Gen. Psychiatr.*, 1974, *31*:189.

Prien, R. F., Caffey, E. M., Jr., and Klett, C. J. The Relationship between Serum Lithium Level and Clinical Response in Acute Manics Treated with Lithium Carbonate. *Br. J. Psychiatr.*, 1972a, *120*:409.

Prien, R. F., Caffey, E. M., Jr., and Klett, C. J. A Comparison of Lithium and Chlorpromazine in the Treatment of Excited Schizo-Affectives. *Arch. Gen. Psychiatr.*, 1972b, *27*:182.

Reilly, E., Halmi, K. A., and Noyes, R. Electroencephalographic Response to Lithium. *Int. Pharmacopsychiatry*, 1973, *8*:208.

Rifkin, A., Quitkin, F., Carrillo, C., Blumberg, A. G., and Klein, D. F. Lithium Carbonate in Emotionally Unstable Character Disorders. *Arch. Gen. Psychiatr.*, 1972, *27*:519.

Schou, M. Special Review: Lithium in Psychiatric Therapy and Prophylaxis. *J. Psychiatr. Res.*, 1968, *6*:67.

Schou, M. Lithium in Psychiatric Therapy—Stocktaking after Ten Years. *Psychopharmacologia*, 1963, *1*:65.

Schou, M., Baastrup, P. C., Grof, P., Weis, P., and Angst, J. Pharmacological and Clinical Problems of Lithium Prophylaxis. *Br. J. Psychiatr.*, 1970, *116*:615.

Sheard, M. H. Effects of Lithium on Human Aggression. *Nature*, 1971, *230*:113.

Shopsin, B., Friedmann, R., and Gershon, S. Lithium and Leukocytosis. *Clin. Pharmacol. Ther.*, 1971, *12*:923.

Shopsin, B., Johnson, G., and Gershon, S. Neurotoxicity with Lithium: Differential Drug Responsiveness. *Int. Pharmacopsychiatr.*, 1970, *5*:170.

Sletten, I. W., and Gershon, S. The Premenstrual Syndrome: A Discussion of Its Pathophysiology and Treatment with Lithium Ion. *Compr. Psychiatr.*, 1966, *7*:197.

Spring, G., Schweid, D., Gray, C., Steinberg, J., and Horwitz, M. A Double-Blind
    Comparison of Lithium and Chlorpromazine in the Treatment of Manic
    States. *Am. J. Psychiatr.*, 1970, *126*:1306.
Thomsen, K., and Schou, M. Renal Lithium Excretion in Man. *Am. J. Physiol.*,
    1968, *215*:823.
Vancaflor, L. Lithium Side Effects and Toxicity: The Clinical Picture, in F. N.
    Johnson (ed.), *Lithium Research and Therapy*. Academic Press, New York,
    1975, pp. 211–216.

CHAPTER 7

Rapid Psychiatric Assessment: Initial and Follow-Up Psychopharmacological Disposition

It has been observed that decisions on psychopharmacotherapy are made frequently on "feel" and inference. Decisions based on vagueries are fraught with failure and responsible for injudicious psychiatric care. Instead, the clinician responsible for initiating and continuing psychopharmacological regimens always must have a clinical, fact-based rationale for prescribing the chosen medication, dosage changes, and duration of prescription. This rationale is based on a clinical approach permitting the clinician to collect psychological data sufficient to arrive at:

1. the identification of potentially psychopharmacologically responsive clinical syndromes (see Chapter 1),
2. the indicated psychotropic drug group and component members of choice,
3. target symptoms and signs to be followed for therapeutic change and evidence of remission,
4. dosage reductions to appropriate maintenance levels, and
5. length of medication treatment.

Furthermore, the clinician, because of usually heavy time commitments, should be able to render these dispositions relatively quickly. The clinical approach discussed in this chapter satisfies these five requirements for rapid psychiatric assessment to determine initial and follow-up psychopharmacologic disposition.

83

INITIAL PSYCHOPHARMACOLOGICAL DISPOSITION

Putting the Patient at Ease

The first step in any medical setting is to place the patient at ease as much as possible. This usually can be accomplished by letting the patient know you are about to collect data that will allow you to help in remedying the problem(s) he or she is experiencing.

Subjective Component

The subjective component consists of specific questions that the examiner asks the patient.

Past psychiatric history. This will include diagnoses and therapeutic success of specific psychotropic agents and a profile of prior compliance with prescribed psychotropic drug regimens.

Psychiatric review of symptoms. This will include the following questions.[1]

1.   How are you sleeping?" If the patient is having sleeping difficul ty, determine the type of problem.
   • Initial sleep disturbance: problem going to sleep, assuming the patient retires at his or her usual time and without preretirement stimulants.
   • Intermittent sleep disturbance: problem of spontaneously awakening during the course of the night, not from noise, pain, voiding impulse, etc.
   • Terminal sleep disturbance: awakening approximately one-half to one-and-a-half hours before the usual time and feeling depressed at or shortly after awakening.
2.   "How are you eating?" Appetite problems themselves are non-specific. For example, appetite decreases or increases may be compatible with either anxiety or depression.
3.   "Have you recently[2] been, or are you currently . . .":

---

[1]Phrasing of questions must be individualized for each patient; the examples noted have been effective, but are merely suggestions.
[2]"Recently" usually means from onset of present illness or interval of time from last psychiatric review of symptoms.

- "nervous?"
- "depressed (sad, blue, feeling hopeless, having crying spells, feeling worthless, etc.)?" If positive response for depression is elicited, determine at what time of day it is most intense: morning, afternoon, evening, no particular change during day, or in response to situations, thoughts, events, etc.
- "suspicious that anyone or anything is out to hurt or harm you?"
- "feeling that people are talking about you behind your back or that things in your environment refer specifically to you?"
- "feeling that you have special or superhuman powers, or an exalted station in life?"
- "feeling guilty or feeling that you have committed some unpardonable sin or crime?"
- "feeling that some power or force is controlling your mind, body, or actions?"
- "feeling that anything is wrong with your body?"
- "feeling that any part of you has expanded in size beyond usual proportions or has split off from the rest of your body?"
- "feeling that you or anything around you seems strange, unreal, or no longer exists?"
- "feeling unusual or atypical concern and preoccupation about religious or philosophical ideas, for example, the cosmos, the higher order of things, the meaning of the universe, etc.?"
- "feeling an incomprehensible dread?"
- "feeling that things or situations you have previously accepted without particular concern have now become significant and/or personally relevant?"
- "hearing voices that no one else is hearing?"
- "seeing visions that no one else is seeing?"
- "feeling sensations on your skin when nothing is producing them?"
- "experiencing smells when nothing is producing them?"
- "experiencing tastes when nothing is producing them?"
- "feeling sensations that your body is being propelled when it isn't?"

4. Check for each of the following cognitive functions in the patient:
- orientation to person, place, and time,
- ability to remember three objects after approximately two minutes,
- ability to repeat six digits forward and four digits in reverse order,

- current president of the United States and/or governor of the patient's state,
- ability to do simple arithmetic, for example, subtracting 5 from 100, 5 from 95, and so on,
- ability to explain such commonly known proverbs as "Don't count your chickens before they hatch" and "Don't cry over spilt milk."

Objective Component (Mental Status Examination)

This phase consists of observations of spontaneous renderings during the clinical interview (before and while the patient answers the questions above).

Motor activity. Observe for overall motility, as well as motor activity in specific parts or functions of the body (including speech), with respect to rate, amplitude, and unusual movements or postures.

Affect. Observe for such expressions as sadness, hostility, elatedness or euphoria, and fearfulness, and note any disparity between the thoughts being expressed and the expression on the patient's face while he or she is expressing them.

Thought processes. Observe for rate, amplitude, continuity, coherence, and so on.

Thought content. Observe for thought content (including any component in the psychiatric review of symptoms) spontaneously rendered.

Level of central nervous system state of consciousness. Observe for altered states of consciousness, for example, stupor or lethargy.

Formulation

After review of Chapter 1 on psychopathology and collection of the data described in the foregoing sections, the clinician should be able to organize the patient's psychological data, determine the presence or absence of one of the psychopharmacologically responsive syndromes, and select the initially indicated psychotropic drug group. The next step is to use the medical review of symptoms by system, past medical history, physical examination, and laboratory data to determine:

1. a presumed or apparent organic origin for the patient's psychiatric presentation (nonfunctional), for which the initial clinical approach of choice would be to remedy the organic cause when possible, and/or

2. whether there are absolute or significant relative contraindications to use of a particular psychotropic agent, and the implications of such findings.

FOLLOW-UP PSYCHOPHARMACOLOGICAL DISPOSITION

The goal of psychopharmacological treatment is remission, not merely chemical restraint or control. Therefore, it is not enough to place the patient on a psychotropic agent regimen and check on progress every now and then. Nor is it acceptable merely to render the patient stuporous with a p.r.n. dosage, without having first fit a p.r.n. mode into a well-conceived and physiologically appropriate regimen. Optimal psychopharmacotherapeutic technique suggests that once the initial assessment is rendered and the patient is placed on a regimen, reassessment should occur *every day* until remission.

There must, then, be a reevaluation format. At least two routines apply. The first is merely following psychopharmacologically responsive *target* symptoms and signs and making therapeutic changes based on these observations. The second is to elicit all subjective and objective data initially obtained (taking only a few moments in most cases) to determine if the original symptoms are present and if new symptoms or signs have appeared after the initial evaluation. This second routine potentially offers the practitioner the opportunity for more complete patient treatment.

Once remission is attained, the clinician should assess the patient at relatively frequent intervals during the plateau-dosage stage and while decreasing dosage to the maintenance level. Naturally, once remission seems assured at the maintenance level, the frequency of reassessment may lessen, depending on the patient's needs. Ideally, however, any patient on psychotropic medications should be seen at least monthly. Whichever follow-up assessment routine is used, it is wise to have some consistent data-recording format to assist the clinician (Levenson & Dunbar, 1977).

Without accurate assessment, it is possible that no decision on patient care, or one not in the patient's best interest, will be made. The acumen with which such decisions are made is based at least in part on the clinical approach. This chapter has offered the practitioner such an approach. Once learned and practiced, it will take most of the guesswork out of psychiatric assessment for psychopharmacological disposition.

It should be noted that psychopharmacotherapy is only one of the treatment interventions for most patients with psychiatric illness. The indicated form of counseling or psychotherapy should accompany medication for the most effective results.

REFERENCES

Levenson, A. J., and Dunbar, P. W. The L-D Trend Oriented Psychiatric Record. *Dis. Nerv. Syst.*, 1977, 38:465.

CHAPTER 8

Practice Review

This chapter is intended to amalgamate and reinforce previously described psychopharmacological data by means of clinical case vignettes, questions, answers, and discussions. Naturally, not every key point can be addressed. It is suggested that the reader first read the cases and attempt to answer the corresponding questions without assistance. After this is done, he or she may advance to the section on answers and discussions. Each answer refers the reader to the appropriate chapter for review.

CASES AND QUESTIONS

Case 1

A 20-year-old man presents with the following clinical complex. A psychiatric review of symptoms shows an initial sleep disturbance, intermittent depression without particular diurnal variation, and a vague sense that those around him have somehow changed in shape and form. Both the balance of his review of symptoms and his mental status examination are within normal limits. His physiological evaluation reveals no absolute or significant relative contraindications to the use of psychotropic medications, nor is there any evidence of a presumed or apparent organic etiology for the psychiatric presentation.

Questions (select the best answer from the choices below).

  1. Which of the following is the patient's diagnosis?
     a. organic brain syndrome
     b. acute schizophrenia

    c.   retarded depression

    d.   incipient schizophrenia

  2. Which of the following is the psychopharmacological class of choice for treatment of this syndrome?

    a.   minor tranquilizers

    b.   tricyclic antidepressants

    c.   lithium carbonate

    d.   major tranquilizers

Case 2

A 17-year-old woman presents with acute schizophrenia. Her physical examination reveals hepatomegaly, and the laboratory evaluation is positive for abnormal liver function tests (SGOT, SGPT, T/D billirubin, and alkaline phosphatase). These are not believed to constitute an organic etiology for the psychiatric presentation. You determine that major tranquilizers are the psychopharmacological class of choice for the acute schizophrenia.

Questions (select the best answer from the choices below).

  1. Your initial clinical approach would be:

    a.   Start the patient on major tranquilizers.

    b.   Hold off prescribing the major tranquilizers until the patient's obvious liver disease is cured.

    c.   Decide that you will never prescribe major tranquilizers for this patient.

    d.   Consult with an internist to see if there are any significant relative physiological contraindications to the prescription of major tranquilizers in this patient.

  2. Assuming you have collected data sufficient to permit the prescription of major tranquilizers, which of the following choices would be the most therapeutically effective for acute schizophrenia?

    a.   trifluoperazine (Stelazine®)

    b.   thioridazine (Mellaril®)

    c.   haloperidol (Haldol®)

    d.   all of the above

  3. From a purely physiological point of view, which of the following choices probably represents the best major tranquilizer to prescribe for this patient?

    a.   chlorpromazine hydrochloride (Thorazine, CPZ)

    b.   mesoridazine (Serantil®)

    c.   fluphenazine (Prolixin®)

    d.   loxapine succinate (Loxitane®)

Case 3

A 43-year-old, obese man presents the following clinical complex. The psychiatric review of symptoms is positive for depression, with no particular diurnal variation, and a paranoid persecutory delusion. The balance of the review is within normal limits. His mental status examination reveals only a significant slowness in overall motility, slowness of verbal and thought production, and a depressed affect. Physiological evaluation fails to reveal any contraindications to the use of psychotropic agents or evidence of an organic etiology for the psychiatric presentation.

Questions (select the best answer from the choices below).

1. The patient's diagnosis is:
   a. acute schizophrenia
   b. anxious depression
   c. organic brain syndrome
   d. retarded depression

2. The initial psychopharmacological treatment of choice for this patient is:
   a. lithium carbonate
   b. minor tranquilizers (e.g., diazepam, Valium®)
   c. major tranquilizers (e.g., chlorpromazine, Thorazine, CPZ)
   d. tricyclic antidepressants (e.g., imipramine, Tofranil®)

3. The usual starting dosage for the agent selected in question 2 is:
   a. 200 mg. per day
   b. 75 mg. per day
   c. 5 mg. per day
   d. 900 mg. per day

4. After the initial psychopharmacological agent produces its primary treatment goal, you find that the patient still retains, on mental status examination, a reduction in overall motility, a depressed affect, and slowness in thought production. No other psychiatric abnormality is present. You would now treat this patient with which of the following psychopharmacological classes?
   a. major tranquilizers (e.g., chlorpromazine, Thorazine, CPZ)
   b. minor tranquilizers (e.g., diazepam, Valium®)
   c. tricyclic antidepressants (e.g., imipramine, Tofranil®)
   d. sympathomimetic amines (e.g., methylphenidate, Ritalin®)

5. The starting dosage of the agent selected in question 4 for this particular patient would be:
   a. 25 mg. per day
   b. 5 mg. per day
   c. 10 mg. per day
   d. 200 mg. per day

Case 4

You see a 37-year-old woman who manifests an acute exacerbation of chronic schizophrenia (two previous occurrences). She has been taking trifluoperazine (Stelazine®) 10 mg. P.O. q̄ a.m. (every morning). The physical examination reveals signs of parkinsonism, which you believe to be caused by the major tranquilizer.

Questions (select the best answer from the choices below).

   1.   The purported primary mechanism of production of the patient's extrapyramidal side effect is believed to be:
   a.   a relative increase in dopamine at the level of the basal ganglia
   b.   a relative decrease in dopamine at the level of the basal ganglia
   c.   a norepinephrine excess at the level of the cerebral cortex
   d.   a deficiency of N-N dimethyltryptamine at the level of the basal ganglia
   2.   You elect to treat the patient's extrapyramidal side effects with benztropine methanesulfonate (Cogentin®). Which of the following best describes this drug's purported mechanism of action?
   a.   lowers dopamine at the level of the basal ganglia
   b.   increases dopamine at the level of the basal ganglia
   c.   lowers norepinephrine at the level of the cerebral cortex
   d.   elevates the level of N-N dimethyltryptamine at the level of the basal ganglia
   3.   You find that benztropine methanesulfonate (Cogentin®) ameliorates the extrapyramidal side effect. Assuming that it had not done so at a therapeutic dosage level, what would have been the next therapeutic intervention in this particular patient?
   a.   Gradually withdraw the patient from the trifluoperazine (Stelazine®).
   b.   Change the patient to a more anticholinergic major tranquilizer.
   c.   Reduce the dosage of the trifluoperazine (Stelazine®).
   d.   Maintain the patient on the trifluoperazine at the same dosage level.
   4.   Assuming that you elect to change the patient to a more anticholinergic major tranquilizer, which of the following agents has the most anticholinergic potential?
   a.   acetophenazine (Tindal®)
   b.   perphenazine (Trilafon®)
   c.   thiothixene (Navane®)
   d.   chlorpromazine (Thorazine, CPZ)

5. Assume you elected to change the patient's major tranquilizer from trifluoperazine hydrochloride (Stelazine®) 10 mg. p.m. q̄ a.m. to thiothixene (Navane®). What then would be the equipotent dosage of thiothixene?

    a.   5 mg. P.O. q.d.
    b.   8 mg. P.O. q.d.
    c.   10 mg. P.O. q.d.
    d.   12 mg. P.O. q.d.

Case 5

A 35-year-old woman has been diagnosed by you as having an acute psychosis manifested by a paranoid grandiose delusion. There is neither an organic etiology for the presentation nor any contraindication to the use of major tranquilizers, the psychopharmacological treatment of choice for this psychiatric state.

Questions (select the best answer from the choices below).

1. Which of the following major tranquilizers would be most therapeutically effective for this patient?

    a.   acetophenazine maleate (Tindal®)
    b.   haloperidol (Haldol®)
    c.   perphenazine (Trilafon®)
    d.   all are approximately equal in therapeutic efficacy.

2. Assuming this were a 65-year-old man with a paranoid grandiose delusional state, your clinical approach would then be:

    a.   Do not treat because of the patient's age and probable illness irreversibility.
    b.   chlorpromazine (Thorazine, CPZ) 200 mg. P.O. q.d.
    c.   haloperidol (Haldol®) 8 mg. P.O. q.d.
    d.   thiothixene (Navane®) 2 mg. P.O. q.d.

3. Assume that the 35-year-old woman in Case 5 had the primary signs of acute schizophrenia. This was a first occurrence for her. Because there were no contraindications, you elected to start her on chlorpromazine 200 mg. P.O. h.s. (*hora somni*, at bedtime). Your clinical approach from that point should ideally be:

    a.   daily psychiatric assessment but no plan to increase her chlorpromazine above 200 mg. per day
    b.   once-a-week psychiatric assessment with plans to stop chlorpromazine as soon as some improvement is noted
    c.   daily psychiatric assessment, increasing the medication in approximately 100 mg. increments until remission is produced

    d.   periodic psychiatric assessment based on the patient's complaining to you that her delusion is not going away

4.   Assuming you produce remission in the 35-year-old woman with acute schizophrenia, what should the next step in your pharmacotherapy be?

    a.   Gradually discontinue the medication.

    b.   Increase the dosage another 100 mg. just for safety's sake.

    c.   Maintain the patient on the lowest dosage required to produce and maintain remission for approximately one month. Then gradually reduce the patient's dosage to maintenance levels with relatively frequent psychiatric assessment preceding each change in regimen.

    d.   Maintain the patient on the lowest dosage required to produce and maintain remission for one year. Then gradually reduce the dosage to maintenance levels with relatively frequent psychiatric assessment preceding each change in regimen.

5.   How long would you probably need to keep this woman on maintenance major tranquilizer treatment for her acute schizophrenia, assuming it was her third occurrence?

    a.   6 months to 1 year

    b.   1 to 2 years

    c.   for the rest of her life

    d.   5 years

6.   How long would you keep the 65-year-old man on maintenance major tranquilizers for his first-occurrence paranoid grandiose delusion?

    a.   for the rest of his life

    b.   1 year

    c.   2 years

    d.   3 years

Case 6

A 40-year-old man presents with the following clinical complex. The psychiatric review of symptoms is positive for an initial and intermittent sleep disturbance, depression (without diurnal variation), and frightening hallucinations. The balance of the subjective inventory is negative for any abnormality. The mental status examination reveals a labile affect, impaired recent memory, and inability to abstract proverbs.

Questions (select the best answer from the choices below).

1.   The most prudent initial clinical approach for this patient is:

    a.   treat initially with major tranquilizers

    b.   treat initially with tricyclic antidepressants

    c.   treat initially with minor tranquilizers, pending pre-prescription evaluation for major tranquilizers

    d.   no pharmacological treatment, pending evaluation of an organic etiology for the patient's clinical presentation

    2.   Assume that you elect to withhold psychopharmacological treatment pending an organic etiological work-up. Your evaluation depicts an irritative focus in the frontotemporal area on electroencephalography. The radionuclide and computerized axial tomographic scans of the brain fail to reveal any specific lesion. The balance of the laboratory investigation is negative. Neurological consultations recommend no further work-up or treatment. You would like to prescribe major tranquilizers because the patient's original clinical complex remains. What is your major concern about the prescription of these agents for this patient?

    a.   They will lower dopamine at the level of the basal ganglia.

    b.   They will depress norepinephrine neuronal activity at the level of the reticular activating system.

    c.   They will lower the seizure threshold.

    d.   They have the potential for causing an allergic hypersensitivity reaction.

    3.   The next therapeutic intervention should be:

    a.   Notify the patient and his wife that it is too dangerous to treat him with major tranquilizers.

    b.   Prescribe minor tranquilizers.

    c.   Prescribe hemodialysis to rid the patient of any toxins that may be causing his psychiatric presentation.

    d.   Consult with the neurology service to determine if a significant reason exists, from a neurological perspective, to avoid treatment with major tranquilizers.

    4.   Assume that, on the basis of the data at hand, you have decided to treat with major tranquilizers. Which of the following agents would you especially want to avoid prescribing?

    a.   acetophenazine (Tindal®)

    b.   haloperidol (Haldol®)

    c.   thioridazine (Mellaril®)

    d.   chlorpromazine (Thorazine, CPZ)

Case 7

A 47-year-old woman presents with the following clinical complex. The psychiatric review of symptoms is positive for an initial and intermittent sleep disturbance, anorexia, and depression worse in the afternoon and evening. The balance of the subjective inventory is within normal limits.

Her mental status examination reveals the following positive findings: stammering speech, almost persistent hand wringing and pacing (she is unable to sit still for longer than 5 or 10 minutes), and inability to concentrate on her problem. The balance of the mental status examination is within normal limits. The laboratory evaluation fails to reveal any organic etiology for the patient's psychiatric presentation or any contraindication to the prescription of psychotropic medications.

Questions (select the best answer from the choices below).

1. The patient's diagnosis is:
   a. retarded depression
   b. anxious depression of moderate to severe intensity
   c. acute hypomania
   d. anxious depression of mild to moderate intensity
2. The psychopharmacological treatment of choice for this patient is:
   a. major tranquilizers
   b. minor tranquilizers
   c. tricyclic antidepressants
   d. lithium
3. After remission is reached, select the next change in the regimen:
   a. Leave the patient on the lowest dose required to produce remission for one week, and then gradually withdraw the patient from the medication, assuming remission still remains.
   b. As soon as remission is attained, gradually reduce the patient's dosage to the maintenance level and continue this level for six months.
   c. As soon as remission is attained, keep the patient on the dosage required to produce remission for approximately one month, and then gradually reduce the dosage to a maintenance dosage level. Continue this level for approximately six months.
   d. When the dosage required to produce remission is known, increase this dosage by 25% to assure maintenance of remission.

Case 8

A 48-year-old man presents a clinical complex compatible with an anxious depression of mild to moderate intensity, accompanied by a nihilistic delusion. There are no contraindications to the prescription of psychotropic drugs.

Questions (select the best answer from the choices below).

1. The initial psychopharmacological regimen of choice for this patient is:

      a.   tricyclic antidepressants
      b.   major tranquilizers and minor tranquilizers
      c.   major tranquilizers alone
      d.   minor tranquilizers alone

   2.   If this is a first occurrence for this clinical complex, how long should the patient be left at the maintenance level of psychotropic medication?

      a.   5 years
      b.   1 to 2 years
      c.   a lifetime
      d.   1 year

Case 9

A 37-year-old, frail, and small-statured woman presents with a retarded depression. There are no contraindications to the prescription of psychotropic medications, and no evidence to support the presence of an organic etiology for the psychiatric presentation.

Questions (select the best answer from the choices below).

   1.   Before prescribing a psychotropic medication, the most important information you need to know first is:

      a.   duration of the retarded depression
      b.   existence of a family history of retarded depression
      c.   whether the retarded depression is accompanied by incipient or manifest schizophrenia, incipient or manifest delusions, or hallucinations
      d.   presence of terminal sleep disturbance

   2.   Assuming you elect to treat with tricyclic antidepressants, specifically imipramine (Tofranil®), what is the most likely starting dosage for this patient?

      a.   75 mg. per day
      b.   50 mg. per day
      c.   25 mg. per day
      d.   100 mg. per day

   3.   Assume you begin a patient who has a tricyclic-antidepressant responsive syndrome on imipramine (Tofranil®) 75 mg. P.O. q̄ h.s. Which of the following best represents an acceptable regimen?

      a.   Allow six weeks after starting dosage before the next regimen change.
      b.   Allow two days after starting dosage and, if there is no improvement, increase the patient's dosage by 75 mg. per day.

c.   Increase the patient's dosage by 25 mg. every day or every other day until remission is produced.

d.   Increase the patient's dosage by 75 mg. per day every day or every other day until remission is produced.

4.   In the absence of age and stature adjustments, the highest dosage of imipramine beyond which improvement probably will not occur but at which the incidence of side effects increases significantly is:

a.   100 mg. per day
b.   200 mg. per day
c.   150 mg. per day
d.   300 mg. per day

Case 10

An 80-year-old woman manifests a retarded depression unaccompanied by incipient or manifest schizophrenia, incipient or manifest delusions, or hallucinations. Her prepsychopharmacological evaluation reveals a history and electrocardiographic determination suggesting arteriosclerotic cardiovascular disease manifested by approximately twice-a-month episodes of angina pectoris, a 1° A-V block, and T-wave inversion; and hypothyroidism shows up on current laboratory evaluation.

Questions (select the best answer from the choices below).

1.   Your initial clinical approach should be:

a.   Begin the patient on tricyclic antidepressants.
b.   Begin the patient on methylphenidate (Ritalin®).
c.   Before initiating psychopharmacotherapy, evaluate and treat the hypothyroidism.
d.   none of the above

2.   It is determined that the hypothyroidism is not considered to be a cause of the patient's psychiatric presentation. You wish to treat the patient with tricyclic antidepressants. What is the next phase of your clinical approach?

a.   Begin the patient on an age-adjusted regimen of tricyclic antidepressants.
b.   Tell the patient and her family that you cannot treat her depression because tricyclic antidepressants are potentially cardiotoxic.
c.   Order a coronary angiogram to determine the extent of cardiovascular arteriosclerosis.
d.   Request an internal medicine consultation to determine (1) if there are any significant physiological contraindications to tricyclic

antidepressants in this patient, and (2) appropriate intraprescription monitoring devices, if approval is given for the use of these agents.

3. You begin the patient on imipramine (Tofranil®) 25 mg. P.O. q̄ h.s., and she complains of drowsiness. Your next step should be:

    a. Discontinue the antidepressant.

    b. Prescribe methylphenidate (Ritalin®).

    c. Reassure the patient that on the basis of the data available, the sedation is probably a side effect of the antidepressant and generally disappears in two to three weeks after initiation of its use.

    d. Switch to a less soporific tricyclic antidepressant, such as doxepin (Sinequan®).

Case 11

A 35-year-old man presents the following clinical complex. A psychiatric review of symptoms is postive for initial and intermittent sleep disturbance. The mental status examination reveals a severe overall hypermotility with pressure of speech, a euphoric affect, and excessively pressured and accelerated thought production with flight of ideas. The balance of the mental status examination fails to reveal any abnormality. There is neither a contraindication to the use of psychotropic medications nor the suggestion of an organic origin for the current clinical presentation.

Questions (select the best answer from the choices below).

    1. The patient's diagnosis is:

        a. acute schizophrenia

        b. organic brain syndrome

        c. anxious depression of moderate to severe intensity

        d. acute mania

    2. The primary psychopharmacological treatment of choice for this syndrome is:

        a. minor tranquilizers

        b. major tranquilizers

        c. lithium carbonate

        d. sleeping medication

    3. For the moderate or severe hypermotility accompanying this syndrome, the initial psychopharmacological regimen of choice is:

        a. lithium and a minor tranquilizer (usually administered via the intramuscular route

        b. lithium and a major tranquilizer

        c. lithium alone

        d. minor tranquilizer

4. Assume that the syndrome noted in Case II is accompanied by a paranoid persecutory delusion. The psychopharmacological regimen of choice is:
    a. lithium and a minor tranquilizer
    b. lithium alone
    c. lithium and a major tranquilizer
    d. major tranquilizers alone
5. Assume that the clinical complex in Case 11 also indicates acute schizophrenia. The psychopharmacological treatment of choice is:
    a. lithium and a major tranquilizer
    b. lithium alone
    c. major tranquilizer alone
    d. minor tranquilizer

Case 12

A 45-year-old man manifests acute mania (without accompanying incipient or manifest schizophrenia, incipient or manifest delusions, hallucinations, or excessive agitation or hypermotility). You elect to treat with lithium carbonate, because the physiological evaluation reveals no contraindications to its use and no evidence of an organic etiology for the patient's psychiatric presentation.
Questions (select the best answer from the choices below).
1. The usual starting dosage of lithium carbonate for this patient would be:
    a. 400 mg. P.O. three times a day
    b. 300 mg. P.O. each morning
    c. 100 mg. P.O. three times a day
    d. 300 mg. P.O. three times a day
2. After the starting dosage is begun, the usual therapeutic regimen with lithium carbonate is:
    a. Do not increase the dosage for approximately one month, then discontinue the agent.
    b. Gradually increase the dosage by 300 mg. every day or every other day until the patient reaches 1800 mg. per day. After one month at this dosage, gradually reduce the dosage to a maintenance level.
    c. Gradually increase the dosage by 300 mg. every day or every other day until the patient attains remission (assuming toxicity does not occur); then, gradually decrease the patient to a maintenance dosage level (usually in 300 mg. decrements).

   d.   After the initial dosage is begun, no further therapeutic intervention is usually necessary.
   3.   The usual therapeutic serum concentration of lithium during the
acute stage of illness is:
       a.   0.8–1.4 mEq./l.
       b.   0.5–1.0 mEq./l.
       c.   0.1–0.5 mEq./l.
       d.   0.8–1.5 mg.%
   4.   The usual therapeutic serum concentration of lithium during the
maintenance phase of treatment is:
       a.   0.2–0.8 mg.%
       b.   0.0–0.8 mg.%
       c.   0.5–1.5 mEq./l.
       d.   0.2–0.8 mEq/l.
   5.   Serum for lithium concentration determination should usually be
collected:
       a.   immediately after the last evening dosage is given
       b.   immediately after the first dose of the day is given
       c.   approximately 8–12 hours after the last dose of the preceding
day is given, or before the first morning dose of the day is given
       d.   approximately three hours after the second dose of the day is
given
   6.   The major indication for a lithium carbonate dosage increase
during the acute stage of illness is:
       a.   a serum lithium concentration not yet in the usual therapeutic
range
       b.   the patient not yet in clinical remission and without clinical
signs of significant side effects or toxicity (verified by serum lithium
determination)
       c.   no history of thyroid disease
       d.   the patient's desire to have the dosage increased

Case 13

A 48-year-old man presents with acute mania accompanied by agitation.
There are no contraindications to the use of psychotropic agents.
Questions (select the best answer from the choices below).
   1.   The usual therapeutic approach for this clinical complex is:
       a.   the acceptable regimen of lithium for the acute mania
       b.   the acceptable regimen of major tranquilizers for anxiety of
moderate to severe intensity

     c.   the acceptable regimen of lithium for the acute mania and an appropriate starting dosage, with increases of major tranquilizers until the agitation is brought under control; then, gradual decrease of major tranquilizers to zero.

     d.   double the usual starting dosage of lithium carbonate

    2.   Assuming that the patient's acute mania is accompanied by delusions and/or hallucinations without an organic etiology, the usual therapeutic approach would be:

     a.   the acceptable lithium regimen for acute mania

     b.   the acceptable lithium regimen for acute mania, in addition to the acceptable regimen of major tranquilizers for delusions and hallucinations

     c.   the acceptable major tranquilizer regimen for acute schizophrenia

     d.   double the usual starting dosage of lithium carbonate

    3.   The primary psychiatric indication(s) for lithium carbonate alone is/are:

     a.   premenstrual tension

     b.   acute mania without incipient or manifest delusions, incipient or manifest schizophrenia, or hallucinations

     c.   acute hypomania without incipient or manifest delusions, incipient or manifest schizophrenia, or hallucinations

     d.   a and c

     e.   b and c

    4.   The primary psychiatric indication for lithium carbonate in maintenance prophylactic states is:

     a.   recurrent premenstrual tension

     b.   recurrent alcohol abuse

     c.   recurrent acute mania or hypomania

     d.   recurrent acute schizophrenia, schizoaffective excited subtype

Case 14

A 60-year-old woman manifests a clinical psychiatric complex compatible with acute hypomania. Her physiological evaluation reveals a history of hypothyroidism; she is now on replacement thyroxin, and is noted still to be hypothyroid on current laboratory evaluation.

Questions (select the best answer from the choices below).

    1.   Your initial therapeutic intervention should be:

     a.   double the thyroid medication

b.   Tell the patient you cannot prescribe lithium because of its effect on the thyroid gland

c.   Request that the internal medicine service evaluate the patient to determine if there are any significant physiological contraindications to the use of lithium carbonate in this patient

d.   none of the above

2.   Assuming that you treat the patient with lithium carbonate, the starting dosage should be:

a.   300 mg. P.O. three times a day
b.   300 mg. P.O. twice a day
c.   300 mg. P.O. four times a day
d.   300 mg. P.O. daily

3.   At 300 mg. P.O. three times a day of lithium carbonate, you note that the patient becomes drowsy and dysarthric. Your next step should be:

a.   Immediately measure the serum lithium level.
b.   Lower the lithium carbonate dosage to 600 mg.
c.   Obtain a neurology consultation.
d.   Obtain an internal medicine consultation.

4.   The risk of dose-related lithium toxicity usually increases at serum concentrations of:

a.   0.5–0.8 mEq./l.
b.   0.8–1.2 mEq./l.
c.   0.2–0.5 mEq./l.
d.   Greater than 1.4 mEq./l.

Case 15

A 32-year-old woman presents the following clinical complex. A psychiatric review of symptoms is positive for an intermittent sleep disturbance and depression that is worse in the afternoon and evening. The balance of the subjective data base is negative for any abnormality. The mental status examination is within normal limits. There are no contraindications to the use of psychotropic medications and no evidence of an organic etiology for the patient's psychiatric presentation.

Questions (select the best answer from the choices below).

1.   This patient's diagnosis is:

a.   anxiety
b.   acute hypomania
c.   retarded depression
d.   anxious depression of mild to moderate intensity

2. The initial psychopharmacological treatment of choice for this
patient is:
    a.   major tranquilizers
    b.   sleeping medication
    c.   tricyclic antidepressants
    d.   minor tranquilizers

Case 16

You prescribe diazepam (Valium®) for a 72-year-old man with an anxious
depression of mild intensity that includes an initial sleep disturbance.
Questions (select the best answer from the choices below).
    1. An appropriate starting dosage of diazepam (Valium®) for this
patient should ideally be:
    a.   5 mg. P.O. twice daily
    b.   5 mg. P.O. three times a day
    c.   1 mg. P.O. every morning and h.s.
    d.   none of the above
    2. After the starting dosage is begun, the major goal of psychophar-
macological treatment is:
    a.   relaxation of the patient's wife
    b.   disappearance of the patient's initial sleep disturbance
    c.   remission of the entire clinical complex
    d.   a decrease in the intensity of the clinical complex
    3. The usual therapeutic regimen for this patient would be:
    a.   discontinuation of minor tranquilizer as soon as you see that
the starting dosage produces some improvement without side effects
    b.   gradual increments in dosage of the agent until remission is
produced, then abrupt discontinuation of the medication
    c.   gradual increase in dosage of the agent until remission is
produced, then gradual decrease of the medication to zero
    d.   gradual increase in dosage of the agent until remission is
produced; continuation of the dosage required to produce remission
for approximately one month; gradual reduction to the maintenance
dosage level, keeping the patient on that level for approximately six
months.

ANSWERS AND DISCUSSIONS

Case 1

Answers.

  1. d (see Chapter 1)
  2. d (see Chapter 3)

Discussion. The criteria for the diagnosis of incipient schizophrenia are important for the following reasons. First, temporal-lobe pathology (e.g., epilepsy) may cause the identical clinical presentation. Note that no organic etiology was present in this case. Second, without psychopharmacological treatment (major tranquilizers), the incipient state may likely progress to manifest schizophrenia, a somewhat more difficult diagnostic entity to treat. Third, it is also important to treat the syndrome, because it carries a relatively high incidence of suicide and homicide (question 1). Regarding the possible psychopharmacological treatment alternatives for incipient schizophrenia, several points are worthy of mention. First, minor tranquilizers are not effective. Tricyclic antidepressants can convert incipient schizophrenia into a manifest state. Lithium carbonate, although not exclusively tested in incipient schizophrenia, has been demonstrated to worsen the clinical status of certain acute schizophrenic states (question 2).

Case 2

Answers.

  1. d (see Chapter 3)
  2. d (see Chapter 3)
  3. d (see Chapter 3)

Discussion. This case, among other things, considers the issue of relative contraindications to the prescription of certain psychotropic agents. Major tranquilizers are the pharmacological treatment of choice for acute schizophrenia; however, this patient presents a physiological problem that could be worsened by these agents. Also, the liver is the major metabolic organ for tranquilizers; this, coupled with the fact that the patient's age suggests immature organ functioning, might indicate special considerations before prescription of major tranquilizers.

Certainly, one should not proceed with the administration of any pharmacological agent that could be affected by, or further affect, impaired liver function. Although preexisting liver disease may not absolutely contraindicate the use of major tranquilizers, it is not prudent to proceed without the benefit of consultation from an internist. However, one should never deny a patient the primary treatment for such a potentially devastating illness as schizophrenia without concrete data sustaining such a decision. In fact, based on the author's experiences with many internal medicine consultations in similar situations, it is often acceptable to administer the psychopharmacological agent (question 1).

From the standpoint of therapy, no major tranquilizer is especially more effective than another, despite the patient's liver problem (question 2). When all psychopharmacological agents have been demonstrated to be equally effective therapeutically, selection of one agent over another will be based on each agent's potential to preserve physiological homeostasis. This issue is addressed in question 3. For example, chlorpromazine, mesoridazine, and fluphenazine all have been implicated in the production of cholestatic jaundice; chlorpromazine is the most commonly implicated, perhaps because of its wider usage. Therefore, one would certainly not prescribe it in this case if there were any alternatives. The alternative is loxapine succinate, metabolized and excreted almost exclusively by the kidneys. Were this agent not available, any one of the other alternatives (except chlorpromazine) could have been prescribed. However, the dosage regimen would need to be lowered appropriately so as not to impose on the hepatic metabolic apparatus. The patient's age certainly commits the physician to age-appropriate changes in regimen. In addition, more-frequent-than-usual liver function tests should be incorporated into the patient-management schema to evaluate homeostasis and, thus, to determine the feasibility of continuing major tranquilizers.

Case 3

Answers.

1. d (see Chapter 1)
2. c (see Chapters 3 and 5)
3. a (see Chapter 3)
4. c (see Chapters 3 and 5)
5. a (see Chapters 3 and 5)

Discussion. The diagnosis is an extremely important consideration from the psychopharmacotherapeutic point of view. Psychomotor retardation in the presence of depression suggests a retarded depression. Any depression may be accompanied by incipient or manifest schizophrenia, incipient or manifest delusions, or hallucinations; this particular case happens to be accompanied by a manifest delusional state (question 1).

Without a clear delineation of this syndrome, an inappropriate psychopharmacological agent or regimen might well be chosen. In this case, the pharmacotherapy must be aimed at the delusion. Likewise, in cases of retarded depression (or any depression for that matter), an accompanying incipient delusion, incipient or manifest schizophrenia, or hallucinations should be the focus of pharmacotherapy. Even though tricyclic antidepressants are the agents of choice for the retarded depression, they are likely to worsen such a clinical syndrome accompanied by one of the above-mentioned psychiatric states, presumably by virtue of their effects on central biogenic amines. Minor tranquilizers have no significant effect on retarded depressions, incipient or manifest schizophrenia, incipient or manifest delusions, or hallucinations. Lithium has been shown to have a possible effect in retarded depressions, but its use is questionable and not superior to tricyclics. The pharmacological treatment of choice in this case, therefore, would be major tranquilizers (question 2).

The usual starting dosage of chlorpromazine, a major tranquilizer, would be approximately 200 mg. per day, whether in one or in divided dosages. Because chlorpromazine is very soporific, it is wise to consider prescribing all or most of it at bedtime. The fact that the patient is obese does not influence the starting dosage. Were the patient slight in stature, a lower starting dosage and smaller increments would be in order (question 3).

Question 4 implies that although the major tranquilizer has created a remission of the delusional state, signs compatible with a retarded depression remain. While the patient remains on the major tranquilizer regimen for the remitted delusional state, a tricyclic antidepressant may now be added to treat the retarded depression. Imipramine is selected (question 4). Because the major tranquilizer administered concomitantly with tricyclic antidepressants can cause a two- to threefold plasma level increase in tricyclic antidepressants, the imipramine must be added in approximately one-third the usual starting dosage, or 25 mg. per day (question 5). The increments of the tricyclic antidepressant would be one-third the usual, and the optimal dosage allowable to produce remission would be approximately one-third the usual. Otherwise, a regimen for tricyclics remains the same as discussed in Chapter 5.

Case 4

Answers.

1. b (see Chapter 3)
2. b (see Chapter 3)
3. b (see Chapter 3)
4. d (see Chapter 3)
5. b (see Chapter 3)

Discussion. Case 4 describes a chronic schizophrenic who manifests an acute exacerbation of this state accompanied by an iatrogenic (treatment-induced) extrapyramidal syndrome, presumably produced by the prescribed major tranquilizer. She is, by usual standards, too young to have idiopathic parkinsonism, and has no past history to suggest a predisposing or other cause. The piperazine phenothiazines, of which trifluoperazine is one, are commonly implicated in the production of this side effect, as are the other more antidopaminergic major tranquilizers, although all have the potential for causing it. With the exception of tardive dyskinesia and some cases of akathisia, these side effects are usually very treatable.

Idiopathic parkinsonism is represented, at least in part, by lowered dopamine at the level of the basal ganglia. Because major tranquilizers are known to exert a portion of their action at the cerebral structures and are believed to block the action of dopamine, it can be seen how they may both lower the central level of this biogenic amine and, hence, produce many of these extrapyramidal side effects (iatrogenic parkinsonism, acute dystonias and dyskinisas, as well as akathisia) (question 1).

Thus, pharmacological treatment of these iatrogenic syndromes should be aimed at elevating the level of this amine. Because there is a relative balance between dopamine and acetylcholine in the brain, any pharmacological agent that lowers acetylcholine will elevate dopamine and, therefore, restore balance of these two neurotransmitters within the basal ganglia. Benztropine methanesulfonate (Cogentin®) is one of several commonly used CNS anticholinergic agents (agents that lower CNS acetylcholine) (question 2). Others include trihexphenidyl (Artane®) and procyclidine (Kemadrin®).

There are at least three other means of treating iatrogenic extrapyramidal syndromes. One may add an agent that promotes direct elevation of dopamine, such as amantadine (Symmetrel®). One may decrease the dosage of the existing major tranquilizer that caused the side effect. Finally, one may switch from the more antidopaminergic major tranquilizers to a more anticholinergic one. Refer to Table 3–2 (Chapter 3) to review the relative anticholinergic potential of the various major tranquilizers. Of course, the patient can be continued on the major tranquilizer producing the extrapyramidal side effect as long as the antiextrapyramidal agent works. Because all of these anticholinergic compounds (e.g., benztropine methanesulfonate) are believed to be equally effective, if a dosage increase is required for the major tranquilizer, with a consequent reappearance of this side effect, then an alternative regimen, either to lower the acetylcholine or create less dopamine blockade, would have to be adopted.

Question 3 raises the issue of treatment strategy for a patient with an episode of a major-tranquilizer-responsive syndrome, such as acute schizophrenia, who fails to respond to the antiextrapyramidal agent. Because these agents were described as being relatively equally effective for such side effects (assuming they are prescribed at therapeutic dosages), an alternative treatment intervention is in order. One certainly would not wish to discontinue the major tranquilizer, for it is the pharmacological treatment of choice in acute schizophrenia; similarly, to reduce the dosage of the current major tranquilizer, without replacing it, would be likely to cause a worsening of the acute schizophrenic state. Furthermore, if a therapeutic dosage of the benztropine methanesulfonate does not ameliorate the syndrome, the practitioner will have to consider changing the patient from the more antidopaminergic major tranquilizer to a more anticholinergic one. Of the choices listed in question 4, chlorpromazine is the most anticholinergic.

The matter of relative equipotence and its effect on required dosage adjustments from one major tranquilizer to another is addressed in question 5. Certainly, if the change is between two equipotent agents, no dosage adjustment is required. However, what dosage of thiothixene is equipotent to trifluoperazine 10 mg. (orally) per day? This can be easily calculated, as follows: a trifluoperazine dosage of 10 mg. per day is equipotent to chlorpromazine 200 mg. per day (trifluoperazine is 20 times more potent than chlorpromazine); thiothixene is 25 times more potent than chlorpromazine; therefore, an equipotent dosage of thiothixene to chlorpromazine 200 mg. per day (and trifluoperazine 10 mg. per day) is 8 mg. per day (8 × 25).

This discussion on relative equipotence focuses on oral administration. To switch from trifluoperazine 10 mg. P.O. per day to the intramuscular dose of thiothixene, one could first compute the equipotent P.O. dosage of thiothixene as discussed above. Because the intramuscular route is three to four times more potent than the P.O. route, one would utilize one-third to one-fourth the P.O. dose for an equipotent intramuscular dosage (one-third of 8 mg. equals approximately 2.5 mg. I.M. per day).

Case 5

Answers.

1. d (see Chapter 3)
2. d (see Chapter 3)
3. c (see Chapter 3)
4. c (see Chapter 3)
5. c (see Chapter 3)
6. b (see Chapter 3)

Discussion. Case 5 further addresses the issue of major tranquilizer regimens. Question 1 reemphasizes the fact that the major tranquilizers listed in Chapter 3 are all equally efficacious from a therapeutic standpoint

Question 2 introduces the age factor in the treatment of major-tranquilizer-responsive syndromes. Regardless of age, these syndromes are potentially treatable to produce remission. The balance of this question refers to age adjustments in dosage. Patients who are younger than approximately 18 years or older than 55 years of age require one-third to one-fourth the usual starting dosage. Because chlorpromazine 200 mg. P.O. per day is the usual nonadjusted starting dosage for the psychiatric state in Case 5, age and equipotence adjustments must be made from that point. Thiothixene 2 mg. P.O. q.d. is the correct answer, since it represents one-fourth of the equipotent dosage of chlorpromazine 200 mg. P.O. q.d.

Question 3 crystallizes portions of the clinical approach. First, the starting dosage for functional syndromes, including incipient or manifest schizophrenia, incipient or manifest delusions, or hallucinations, is the same: chlorpromazine 200 mg. P.O. per day or the equipotent dosage for another major tranquilizer or route of administration. Once this dosage is begun, the treatment goal is remission. En route to this end point, the patient should receive daily psychiatric assessment and approximately 100 mg. increases of chlorpromazine every day or every other day (or the equivalent if another agent is used). Naturally, these values are not age- or stature-adjusted and would have to be so. Anything short of this goal is not in the best interests of the patient, barring physiological complications.

Question 4 is concerned with continuation of the major-tranquilizer regimens in any of the aforementioned psychiatric states. Briefly stated, the patient should be left on the lowest dosage required to produce remission for approximately one month, and then gradually decreased by approximately one-fifth to one-sixth of this dosage every several days to a maintenance level (usually one-third to one-fourth of the lowest dosage required to produce remission). It must be underscored that the maintenance level is just that—the lowest dosage required to maintain remission. In this determination, however, the clinician should be guided by the one-third to one-fourth rule, barring any psychological or physiological problems. Too large a reduction in dosage may cause an exacerbation of the acute psychiatric illness. Never increase the medication without concrete indications, for which "safety's sake" does not qualify. Discontinuing the medication prematurely after remission considerably increases the risk of exacerbation.

Question 5 tests for the length of time, considering the variables of illness and chronicity, the patient ideally should remain on maintenance with major tranquilizers. For acute psychiatric states that include incipient or first-occurrence schizophrenia, incipient or manifest delusions, or hallucinations, the length of maintenance pharmacological treatment is approximately one year. Because major tranquilizers have been found to substantially reduce recurrence in schizophrenia, more than one occurrence usually requires a lifetime of maintenance treatment. Lifetime major tranquilizer treatment is seriously considered for other states, should they recur, but such decisions should be based on individual patient needs. Question 6 raises an additional factor in length of maintenance treatment: the effect of age. Age should have no bearing on this decision, short of any physiological problem that might militate against continuation of the pharmacotherapy. Regardless of age, length of maintenance treatment is dependent on disease state, recurrence, and the significance of side effects or complications.

Unless significant side effects or complications arise, major tranquilizers should never be abruptly withdrawn. To do so involves a risk of withdrawal effects, as well as a worsening of clinical psychiatric status.

Case 6

Answers.

1. d (see Introduction, Chapters 1 and 3)
2. c (see Chapter 3)
3. d (see Introduction, Chapters 1 and 3)
4. d (see Chapter 3)

Discussion. This case reviews the question of psychopharmacological treatment in the presence of symptoms and signs compatible with a psychiatric state having a presumed organic etiology. It specifically deals with major tranquilizers; however, in general, the concept addressed is applicable to all psychotropic drug groups. The treatment of choice for a psychiatric state with presumed or apparent organic etiology is ideally the delineation and reversal of the etiological factor(s). If a physiological evaluation fails to reveal a cause clearly, or if a cause is identifiable but believed to be irreversible, or if in the process of the evaluation the patient's psychiatric states pose a potential threat to him or others, then psychopharmacological treatment appropriate to the indicated syndrome can be considered. However, this treatment ideally should not proceed without clearance from the nonpsychiatric specialists involved.

Question 2 reviews the theory of relative contraindications. Specifically, the organic work-up reveals a possible seizure focus. Because the evaluation fails to reveal any reversible lesion, and consultants do not recommend any further evaluation or treatment, the decision must be made as to whether or not major tranquilizers should be prescribed; they have been shown to lower the seizure threshold. As you feel they are indicated for the patient's clinical psychiatric syndrome, but are concerned about their potential effect on the patient's central nervous system status, it is wise to consult a neurologist or neurosurgeon, who will evaluate the neurological advisability of major tranquilizer administration and the required special regimen changes and precautions (question 3).

Question 4 tests for the selection of the specific major tranquilizer, considering side effects. Because chlorpromazine has been implicated in lowering the seizure threshold more commonly than the other major tranquilizers, it should not be used for this patient.

Case 7

Answers.

1. b (see Chapter 1)
2. a (see Chapters 3 and 4)
3. c (see Chapter 3)

Discussion. This case describes an anxious depression. The diagnosis rests on the delineation of certain symptoms and/or signs (unlike the retarded depression, which is diagnosed entirely from an objective data base: the mental status examination). An anxious depression is worse in the afternoon or evening, it lacks a particular diurnal variation, or occurs in response to situations, and it is accompanied by an initial or intermittent sleep disturbance and symptoms or signs of anxiety. As with retarded depressions, anxious depressions can be accompanied by incipient or manifest schizophrenia, incipient or manifest delusions, or hallucinations. They may also have an organic etiology.

The class of psychotropic agents to be prescribed depends on a correct assessment of the depression's intensity. Naturally, except in very mild or very severe cases, it may be difficult to assess the syndrome's severity accurately. A decision may sometimes be facilitated by the presence or absence of other data. For example, minor tranquilizers are the initial psychopharmacological class of choice in anxious depressions of mild to moderate intensity, without accompanying incipient or manifest schizophrenia, incipient or manifest delusions, or hallucinations. But any anxious depression accompanied by one of the latter syndromes requires major tranquilizers as the initial treatment of choice. In the absence of these accompanying states, or in what appear to be more severe states of anxious depression, minor tranquilizers in age-appropriate dosages may be tried first, with a change in regimen to major tranquilizers if needed (questions 1 and 2).

Question 3 reclarifies the therapeutic regimen in anxious depressions unaccompanied by incipient or manifest schizophrenia, incipient or manifest delusions, or hallucinations. Briefly stated, as soon as the starting dosage is determined, the dosage of the major tranquilizer is gradually increased until remission. The patient is kept on that dosage for approximately one month, barring any unforeseen physiological or psychological complications. The dosage is then gradually reduced by approximately one-fifth to one-sixth of the remission-producing dosage every several days, to a maintenance dosage level that usually amounts to approximately one-third to one-fourth of the lowest dosage level required to produce and maintain remission. The patient remains on this maintenance regimen for approximately six months.

Case 8

Answers.

1.   c (see Chapter 3)
2.   d (see Chapter 3)

Discussion.   This case further elaborates the psychopharmacological treatment approach to anxious depressions. Here, intensity of the syndrome is *not* the key issue in selecting a particular psychotropic drug class; the symptoms and/or signs accompanying the anxious depression are the significant element in planning the initial pharmacological treatment for this patient. Again, regardless of intensity, major tranquilizers are the initial psychopharmacological treatment of choice for any syndrome (including anxious depressions) exhibiting incipient or manifest schizophrenia, incipient or manifest delusions, or hallucinations (question 1).

Question 2 addresses the length of maintenance of psychopharmacological treatment. Specifically, anxious depressions, unaccompanied by one or more of the syndromes mentioned in the discussion of question 1, require approximately six months of maintenance treatment. With one of these syndromes accompanying the depression, the length of maintenance is approximately one year. This approach applies to first-occurrence states. If the state recurs after termination of the maintenance period, lifetime maintenance is considered in regimen planning.

Case 9

Answers.

1. c (see Chapters 1, 3 and 5)
2. c (see Chapter 5)
3. c (see Chapter 5)
4. d (see Chapter 5)

Discussion. This case offers evidence to support the diagnosis of a retarded depression, normally a tricyclic-antidepressant-responsive syndrome. However, one should avoid tricyclic antidepressant pharmacological treatment for retarded depression accompanied by either an incipient or manifest schizophrenia, incipient or manifest delusions, or hallucinations, because tricyclic antidepressants are believed to elevate central levels of biogenic amines (specifically dopamine and serotonin), implicated in the production or worsening of these psychiatric states. Therefore, before prescribing tricyclics, one must verify the presence or absence of such agent-sensitive psychiatric states. Duration of the retarded depression, family history, and presence of a terminal sleep disturbance are not significant considerations in either the diagnosis of a retarded depression or selection of the psychotropic drug class (question 1).

Question 2 is concerned with adjusting dosages in response to small stature. Generally, this requires the use of approximately one-third of the usual starting dosage. In the case of imipramine (Tofranil®), the usual nonadjusted starting dosage is 75 mg. P.O. per day (administered either once a day or in divided dosages). Because this patient is described as being "frail and small statured," the stature-adjusted dosage of this particular tricyclic antidepressant is 25 mg. per day.

Once the patient is begun on the starting dosage, her dosage should be increased in 25 mg. increments (question 3) until remission is produced, a dosage theory common to all psychopharmacologically responsive clinical entities. Seventy-five milligram increases per day would be excessive, increasing the risk of unduly taxing physiological homeostasis. Allowing six weeks after regimen initiation to increase the dosage is not satisfactory, for it clearly and unnecessarily prolongs time of recovery.

Question 4 raises a key issue. All too often, problems exist with suboptimal therapeutic outcome with tricyclics. This is usually for three major reasons: inaccurate diagnosis, inappropriately low dosages, and insufficient length of time allowed for therapeutic response after the highest dose is reached (usually seven to 10 days are required). However, it is important to note two factors. First, dosages above 300 mg. per day, or the equivalent of another antidepressant, have been shown to be no more effective, and second, they significantly increase the risk of untoward reactions. Therefore, assuming the diagnosis and dosage regimen are correct, lack of remission generally requires reassessment and an alternative treatment.

Case 10

Answers.

1. c (see Chapter 5)
2. d (see Chapter 5)
3. c (see Chapter 5)

Discussion.   The answer to question 1 requires recognition of a psychiatric state (including depressions) that potentially has an organic cause. The initial clinical intervention in such a state should be treatment of the hypothyroidism and assessment of the effect of its treatment on the psychiatric state. Psychopharmacotherapeutic intervention should be withheld pending this evaluation.

If reversal of the hypothyroidism has no significant effect on the retarded depression, then psychopharmacological intervention—the use of tricyclic antidepressants—becomes the primary consideration. In this particular case, a significant relative contraindication to their use arises. The patient has a history of active cardiovascular disease, which could be worsened by tricyclics. An internist should be consulted, before tricyclics are prescribed, to evaluate the advisibility of their use in treatment. Frequently, the internist will approve an antidepressant regimen, so it is not prudent to rule out such treatment beforehand; nor is it appropriate to perform an extensive cardiovascular evaluation in the absence of the internist (question 2).

The question of commonly occurring side effects (drowsiness) must be considered as significant in most cases (the soporific potential of the various tricyclics is presented in Chapter 5). Sedation or drowsiness as a side effect is not a contraindication to their continued use, except in cases when an altered state of central nervous system consciousness exists of the patient's safety is threatened. Because this side effect is usually self-limited, neither the addition of a central nervous stimulant nor a change to a less soporific agent seems indicated. At any rate, doxepin (Sinequan®) is not less soporific than imipramine (Tofranil®) (answer to question 3). If the sedation does not disappear after two to three weeks, or if it disturbs the patient, the larger part of the dosage (or the total dosage) may be administered at bedtime. If this regimen change still fails to improve patient satisfaction, then a less soporific agent may be prescribed.

Case 11

Answers.

1. d (see Chapters 1 and 6)
2. c (see Chapter 6)
3. b (see Chapter 3 and 6)
4. c (see Chapters 3 and 6)
5. c (see Chapters 3 and 6)

Discussion. Question 1 addresses the criteria for the diagnosis of acute mania. It should be remembered that the key criteria for diagnosis are usually based on objective data (mental status examination). The diagnosis of acute schizophrenia is based on the presence of the primary Bleulerian signs. Organic brain syndromes are manifested by a labile or blunted affect; impaired recent memory; partial or total disorientation to person, place, or time; impaired digit retention or intellectual function; or inability to reason abstractly. Although there is hypermotility in an anxious depression, it is compatible with anxiety. Such signs as hand wringing, stuttering, or stammering are not particularly suggestive of acute mania or hypomania. Furthermore, anxiety states do not generally manifest pressure of speech or thought, or euphoria—especially not anxiety accompanied by depression.

A pharmacological treatment of choice for acute mania is lithium carbonate. Some clinicians and researchers feel that major tranquilizers are effective for this syndrome, but not necessarily more so than lithium. The apparent effectiveness of the major tranquilizers may result from their control of the manic hypermotile state or from an inaccurate initial diagnosis. Sleeping medications, possibly helpful at first, are not antimanic agents. Presumably, when the acute mania begins to respond to lithium, the accompanying sleep problem will no longer remain a significant issue (question 2).

Because it takes approximately six to 10 days for the initiation of lithium-induced clinical improvement, manic hypermotility or agitation may require concomitant major tranquilizer treatment. The nonadjusted major tranquilizer regimen usually begins with approximately 100–200 mg. per day of chlorpromazine, or the equivalent dosage for another agent, followed by gradual increase to the point of control. In six to 10 days after initiation of lithium therapy, when the hypermotile state appears resolved or nearing resolution, the major tranquilizer may be withdrawn gradually, barring any unforeseen problems (question 3).

Lithium is not conclusively antidelusional (although antimanic), but major tranquilizers *are* (although not conclusively antimanic); thus, a regimen of lithium and major tranquilizers is in order for acute mania accompanied by incipient or manifest delusions (or hallucinations). Each psychotropic-agent regimen is established as if the syndromes were being treated separately (question 4). If acute mania or hypomania is accompanied by incipient or manifest schizophrenia, the syndrome should be considered a schizophrenic state; the thrust of the pharmacotherapy should be aimed at the schizophrenic process. This is because lithium has not been demonstrated conclusively to be effective in schizophrenic states, whereas major tranquilizers have.

Case 12

Answers.

1. d (see Chapters 3 and 6)
2. c (see Chapter 6)
3. a (see Chapter 6)
4. d (see Chapter 6)
5. c (see Chapter 6)
6. b (see Chapter 6)

Discussion. Because this case evinces no need for dosage adjustments (e.g., age, stature, significant heart or renal disease), 300 mg. P.O. three times a day appears acceptable (question 1). The same concept of dosage regimens applying to the other psychotropic drug groups applies to lithium. Generally speaking, the goal of psychopharmacological treatment is the attainment and maintenance of remission. After the patient is begun on the starting dosage of lithium carbonate, the dosage is gradually increased (usually in 300 mg. increments) every day or every other day until remission is attained. With appearance of significant side effects, however, a dosage decrease might be indicated. Clinical psychiatric assessment is the main guideline before each dosage change. Serum lithium determinations are useful to ascertain attainment of the therapeutic range, but primarily should be used either to forestall or to corroborate the presence of dose-related side effects. Unlike the procedure for other psychopharmacological classes, however, once the lowest remission-producing dosage is determined, the dosage should gradually be reduced to the maintenance level (usually one-third to one-fourth of the remission-producing dosage). This is because the central nervous system is believed to use less lithium as the clinical condition improves. If reduction of the lithium dosage were not started immediately at remission, there would ordinarily be a rather rapid increase in the serum lithium concentration, hence an increased risk of toxicity (questions 2 and 6).

The approximate therapeutic range of serum lithium concentration during the acute stage of illness is 0.8–1.4 mEq./l. Above this range there is an increased risk of side effects, and below it there is a decreased chance of a successful therapeutic outcome (question 3). Because lithium has been found to be prophylactic against recurrent hypomania and mania, and because there is a correlation between the clinical state of prophylaxis and the serum lithium level, this determination can be helpful in management of the maintenance state. This generally occurs in the 0.2–0.8 mEq./l. range. However, the patient by no means needs to be either at the upper or lower limit of this spectrum. It is not uncommon to find a patient in maintenance remission at the 0.2–0.4 mEq./l. level or unstable at the 0.6–0.8 mEq/l. level. It should, therefore, be underscored that determination of clinical state is an individual matter, and serum lithium concentrations, although extremely helpful, are not the only determinant (question 4). As with the acute stage of illness, clinical assessment in the interview situation must be the major determinant of maintenance.

Collection time for the serum lithium determination should ideally be consonant with the standardization methodology for the test. Values are obtained and correlated with clinical status on the flame photometer eight to 12 hours after the last dose of the day. Since this timing generally falls around early morning the next day, standard clinical practice usually suggests phlebotomy before the first morning dose of the day (question 5).

Case 13

Answers.

1. c (see Chapters 3 and 6)
2. b (see Chapters 3 and 6)
3. e (see Chapter 6)
4. c (see Chapter 6)

Discussion. Infrequently, agitation or excessive hypermotility accompanies acute mania and sometimes acute hypomania. This agitation or hyperactivity is usually lithium-responsive (as a part of the mania or hypomania), but there is a six to 10 day lag time for the lithium to initiate therapeutic improvement. Lithium alone may be insufficient to control this excessive hyperactivity until adequate tissue levels have been attained. Doubling the dosage of lithium to control the agitation places the patient at greater risk of toxicity (question 1). During the interim period, psychopharmacological control with major tranquilizers often is required for the hypermotility or agitation in the more extreme states. The usual major tranquilizer regimen in these cases involves the use of a more soporific agent, such as chlorpromazine, begun at approximately 100–200 mg. per day, or the equivalent for another agent (age- and stature-adjusted). The dosage of the major tranquilizer is increased in approximately 50–100 mg. increments every day or every other day until agitation or hypermotility is approaching control. If at the end of six to 10 days therapeutic results are noted, the major tranquilizer may be withdrawn gradually.

Were the acute mania accompanied by an incipient or manifest delusion or hallucination, a major tranquilizer along with lithium would be indicated. However, rather than being an interim regimen, major tranquilizers would be started at approximately 200 mg. per day for chlorpromazine or the equivalent dosage for another agent, with further dosage adjustments as indicated. The dosage would be increased every day or every other day by 100 mg. of chlorpromazine, or the equivalent until remission occurred. Continuation of the remission-producing dosage for approximately one month would be followed by gradual decrease to a maintenance level, with a maintenance time of one year.

Lithium has not been shown conclusively to be antidelusional or antihallucinatory and, therefore, should be prescribed by itself for this patient. Major tranquilizers are antidelusional and antihallucinatory, but not conclusively antimanic or more efficacious than lithium and, therefore, not necessarily useful as the sole agent in this case. Delusions and/or hallucinations are not, by themselves, compatible with acute schizophrenia. Therefore, treatment for the latter syndrome is not indicated (question 2).

Premenstrual tension, alcoholism, epileptoid personality disorders, and depressions have not been unequivocally demonstrated to be lithium responsive states. Mania and hypomania have, both acutely and prophylactically (questions 3 and 4).

Case 14

Answers.

1. c (see Chapter 6)
2. d (see Chapter 6)
3. a (see Chapter 6)
4. d (see Chapter 6)

Discussion. Lithium can exacerbate hypothyroidism. Therefore, before prescribing it for a patient with this disorder, it is prudent to consult with an internist. This consultation will aid in determining if the agent will disrupt physiological homeostasis so severely that the disadvantages of its administration outweigh the advantages. Hypothyroidism usually does not entirely preclude use of lithium, so, unless the consultant advises against it, there is no need to reject this treatment entirely. It is not wise to double the patient's thyroid replacement; this is not a usual procedure, and should be handled by an expert in this disorder (question 1).

As there is an age limitation, one-third of the usual starting dosage is the rule. Therefore 300 mg. P.O. q.d. is appropriate (question 2).

Question 3 raises the issue of dose-related side effects. When these are suspected, the serum lithium level should be tested immediately to corroborate. Although side effects can and should be corroborated by serum determination, their mere presence should be sufficient indication to lower the dosage of lithium, watching for reversal of the untoward reaction (questions 3 and 4).

Case 15

Answers.

1. d (see Chapters 1 and 4)
2. d (see Chapter 4)

Discussion. The correct diagnosis is anxious depression. Once again, the intensity or severity is sometimes difficult to assess. However, choice d is the best possible alternative for question 1. If the intensity were more extreme, there would normally be evidence of anxiety or depression on the mental status examination (described as being within normal limits in this case). In making a diagnosis of anxious depression irrespective of intensity, it is important to remember that depression that is worse in the afternoon or evening, without any particular diurnal variation, or in response to situations, or accompanied by an initial or intermittent sleep disturbance, or accompanied by anxiety (subjective or objective) is compatible with this state. The presence of depression rules out a pure anxiety state as well as hypomania (especially in the absence of elation or euphoria). Retarded depressions are manifested by depression in the presence of psychomotor retardation, the latter being absent in this patient (question 1).

Minor tranquilizers are the psychopharmacological agents of choice in anxious depressions of mild to moderate intensity. Because major tranquilizers are potentially more toxic, they should usually be avoided in the less severe states. Tricyclic antidepressants have as their main psychiatric indication retarded depressions. Sleeping medications (hypnotics) are not directly anxiolytic or antidepressant in their effects. Furthermore, the clinical approach to anxiety- or depression-induced sleep disturbances is reversal of the anxiety and/or depression, the insomnia usually being ameliorated as the causative processes improve (question 2).

Case 16

Answers.

1. c (see Chapter 4)
2. c (see Chapter 4)
3. d (see Chapter 4)

Discussion. Age adjustment of the starting dosage of diazepam (Valium®) is indicated for this 72-year-old patient. The most common causes of side effects (e.g., sedation, paradoxical agitation, ataxia, organic brain syndrome) tend to be excessive dosage or regimens not titrated in smaller increments. The usual starting dosage of this agent is approximately 5 mg. P.O. per day. Age adjustment, or one-third to one-fourth of the usual starting dosage, suggests 2 mg. P.O. per day (or 1 mg. P.O. twice daily) (question 1).

Once again, the goal of drug treatment is remission. Minor tranquilizers are no exception. After the starting dosage is begun, the minor tranquilizer regimen for the patient described in Case 16 might be as follows: 1–2-mg. increments every other day until remission is reached; continuation on the lowest remission-producing dose for approximately one month; then gradual reduction of this dosage in 1–2-mg. decrements every several days to a maintenance level (usually one-third to one-fourth of the remission-producing dosage); continuation at the maintenance level for approximately six months, barring any unforeseen physiological or psychological complications. Without an emergent cause, an abrupt discontinuation of the medication, which might result in a withdrawal reaction, should be avoided. Naturally, psychiatric assessment should not only precede the regimen initiation, but also every dosage change. Remission indicates amelioration of the acute symptoms and signs of the clinical complex, not merely portions of it or solely a reduction in intensity (questions 2 and 3).

Index

Index

125